Heart Sounds

made Incredibly Easy!®

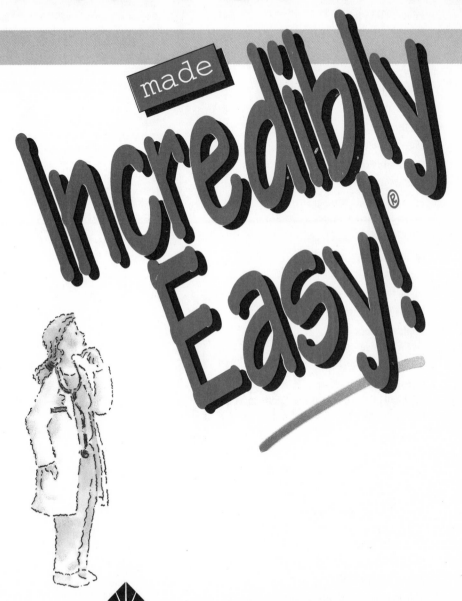

LIPPINCOTT WILLIAMS & WILKINS
A **Wolters Kluwer** Company

Philadelphia • Baltimore • New York • London
Buenos Aires • Hong Kong • Sydney • Tokyo

Staff

Executive Publisher
Judith A. Schilling McCann, RN, MSN

Editorial Director
David Moreau

Clinical Director
Joan Robinson, RN, MSN

Senior Art Director
Arlene Putterman

Art Director
Mary Ludwicki

Electronic Project Manager
John Macalino

Editorial Project Manager
Jaime Stockslager Buss

Clinical Project Manager
Minh N. Luu, RN, BSN, JD

Editors
Diane Labus, Brenna H. Mayer, Julie Munden,
Liz Schaeffer, Gale Thompson

Clinical Editors
Lisa M. Bonsall, RN, MSN, CRNP;
Mary Perrong, RN, MSN, CRNP, APRN,BC, CPAN

Copy Editors
Kimberly Bilotta (supervisor), Scotti Cohn, Shana
Harrington, Dorothy P. Terry, Pamela Wingrod

Designers
Lynn Foulk

Illustrator
Bot Roda

Digital Composition Services
Diane Paluba (manager), Joyce Rossi Biletz
Manufacturing
Patricia K. Dorshaw (director), Beth J. Welsh

Editorial Assistants
Megan L. Aldinger, Tara L. Carter-Bell ,
Linda K. Ruhf

Indexer
Barbara Hodgson

HRTSIE010904—041206

Heart sounds made incredibly easy.
        p. ; cm.
    Includes bibliographical references and index.
        1. Heart—Sounds. 2. Auscultation.
    I. Lippincott Williams & Wilkins.
    [DNLM: 1. Heart Sounds—physiology—Handbooks.
    2. Heart Auscultation—methods—Handbooks.
    3. Heart Diseases—diagnosis—Handbooks.
    4. Heart Murmurs—Handbooks. WG 39 H4348 2005]

RC683.5.A9H436 2005
616.1'207544—dc22
ISBN13 978-1-58255-358-0
ISBN10 1-58255-358-0 (alk. paper)   2004006363

Contents

Contributors and consultants

Shari A. Regina Cammon, RN, MSN, CCRN
Clinical Risk Management and Safety Surveillance Associate
Merck & Co., Inc.
West Point, Pa.

Deborah A. Hanes, RN, MSN, CNS, CRNP
Nurse Practitioner, Cardiothoracic Surgery
The Cleveland Clinic Foundation

David J. Hartman, RN, MSN, CRNP
Nurse Practitioner
University of Pennsylvania
Philadelphia

Gary R. Jones, RN, MSN, FNP-C
Family Nurse Practitioner
Heart Care & Surgical Associates
Joplin, Mo.

Valerie Mignatti, RN, BSN
Clinical Cardiovascular Nurse
University of Pennsylvania Medical Center
Philadelphia

Mary A. Stahl, RN, MSN, APRN,BC, CCRN
Clinical Nurse Specialist
Saint Luke's Hospital
Kansas City, Mo.

Lei Xi, MD
Instructor of Medicine
Virginia Commonwealth University
Richmond, Va.

Foreword

Despite a reduction in heart-related morbidity and mortality in the last few decades, cardiovascular disease remains the leading cause of death in the United States today. As technology in the field advances, it's imperative that nurses remain astute in their physical assessment skills. Because the value of inspection, percussion, and palpation is limited to some degree in the assessment of heart sounds, auscultation remains the mainstay of the physical assessment of patients with cardiovascular disorders. Two necessary ingredients for auscultation of heart sounds are a good stethoscope and a fundamental knowledge of both technique and clinical significance.

Heart Sounds Made Incredibly Easy is a good resource for establishing the knowledge base required for acute auscultation. This one-of-a-kind book assists the learner in sharpening cardiac auscultation skills in a user-friendly, fun approach. It helps hone the proficiency necessary to develop a systematic approach for auscultation of heart sounds that will help you avoid missing key assessments. The accompanying audio CD helps teach how to isolate sounds, concentrate on one sound at a time, and listen selectively. Knowing to pause between cycles, not to rush, and understanding that a novice clinician can't hear everything at once are just some of the secrets to mastering the skill and art of auscultation of heart sounds that are offered in this distinctive reference.

In *Heart Sounds Made Incredibly Easy*, you'll find everything you need to refine your auscultation skills—all in a handy paperback format that's readily available in a busy clinical setting. Logically organized, this unique reference starts with understanding the basic structure and physiology of the heart, the electrical conduction system, and the vascular system; obtaining a detailed health history to correlate with the physical assessment; reviewing the basics of a stethoscope; and outlining both traditional and alternative auscultative techniques. Next, heart sounds are covered extensively, starting with review of the first and second heart sounds, third and fourth heart sounds, ejection sounds (both diastolic and systolic), systolic and diastolic murmurs, continuous murmurs and, finally, prosthetic heart valve sounds. The book concludes with a discussion of cardiovascular conditions and their related heart sounds. It even has an appendix that correlates auscultation findings with common cardiovascular disorders.

Like the other texts in the *Incredibly Easy* series, this book uses several approaches to make learning enjoyable and informative. Here are just some of its fun-filled features:
• An accompanying CD that allows the reader to hear the heart sounds described in the text. The CD can be used with the book or as a stand-alone learning aid.
• Learning objectives at the beginning of each chapter and *Quick quizzes* at the end help the reader gauge learning.

• Short paragraphs and bulleted information encourage rapid understanding of the content.

• More than 200 illustrations highlight cardiovascular anatomy, physiology, and pathophysiology, optimizing understanding of auscultation locations.

In addition to all this, attractive logos articulate vital information to the reader, such as:

Now hear this! — tips for enhancing auscultation skills

Location, location, location — hints on the best placement for the stethoscope

Ages and stages — age-related differences in heart sounds

Memory joggers — mnemonics and other learning aids that assist the reader in grasping critical information.

Heart Sounds Made Incredibly Easy is one book that I'll certainly keep in my collection for quick review. It's a useful text for both the novice and the expert clinician. I hope you'll like the series and this book as much as I do.

Leslie Davis, RN, MSN, ANP, CS
Clinical Assistant Professor
University of North Carolina
School of Nursing/School of Medicine
Division of Cardiology
Chapel Hill

Anatomy and physiology

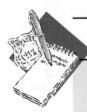

Just the facts

In this chapter, you'll learn:

♦ heart structures and their functions

♦ the heart's conduction system

♦ blood flow through the heart and body.

A look at the cardiovascular system

The cardiovascular system (sometimes referred to as the *circulatory system*) consists of the heart, blood vessels, and lymphatics. A powerful, muscular organ, the heart pumps blood to all organs and tissues of the body. The vascular network—comprising the arteries and veins—carries blood throughout the body, keeps the heart filled with blood, and maintains blood pressure. This chapter discusses each part of this critical system.

Heart structure

The heart consists of cardiac and smooth muscles. On average, an adult's heart is about 4¾″ (12 cm) long from the top (commonly referred to as the *base*) to the bottom (commonly referred to as the *apex*) and 3⅛″ (8 cm) wide at its widest point—or about the size of a closed fist. The heart gradually increases in size from infancy through early adulthood and is usually slightly larger in men than in women.

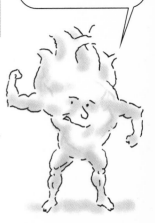

Don't let my size fool you. I'm a powerful muscle that pumps blood to all organs and tissues of the body.

Where the heart calls home

The heart is situated beneath the sternum in the mediastinum (the cavity between the lungs), between the second and sixth ribs. In most people, the heart lies obliquely, with its right side below and almost in front of the left. Because of its oblique angle, the heart's base is located at its upper right, and its pointed apex is located at its lower left. The apex is the point of maximal impulse, where heart sounds are the loudest.

A heart divided

A sac called the *pericardium* surrounds the heart, and a thin wall (called the *septum*) divides the heart into right and left sides. Each side is further divided into two chambers (an atrium and a ventricle). The heart also contains four valves (two atrioventricular [AV] and two semilunar valves). (See *Inside the heart.*)

The pericardium

The pericardium is a two-layer fibroserous sac that surrounds the heart and the roots of the great vessels (those vessels that enter and leave the heart). It consists of the fibrous pericardium and the serous pericardium.

Fibrous fits freely

The fibrous pericardium, composed of tough, white fibrous tissue, fits loosely around the heart, protecting it.

Serous is smooth

The serous pericardium, the thin, smooth inner portion of the pericardium, has two layers:
• The *parietal* layer lines the inside of the fibrous pericardium.
• The *visceral* layer adheres to the surface of the heart.

Room to move

Between the fibrous and serous pericardium is the pericardial space. This space contains pericardial fluid that lubricates the surfaces of the space and allows the heart to move easily during contraction.

Inside the heart

Within the heart lie four chambers (two atria and two ventricles) and four valves (two atrioventricular and two semilunar valves). A system of blood vessels carries blood to and from the heart.

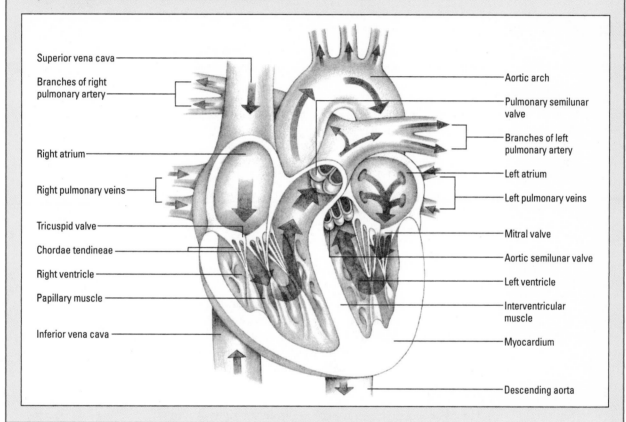

The wall

The wall of the heart consists of three layers:

✌ The *epicardium*, the outer layer (and the visceral layer of the serous pericardium), is made up of squamous epithelial cells overlying connective tissue.

✌ The *myocardium*, the middle layer, forms most of the heart wall. It has striated muscle fibers that cause the heart to contract.

The *endocardium*, the heart's inner layer, consists of endothelial tissue with small blood vessels and bundles of smooth muscle.

> Instead of bricks and mortar, my wall consists of the epicardium, myocardium, and endocardium.

The chambers

The heart contains four hollow chambers: two atria (the plural form of the word *atrium*) and two ventricles.

Upstairs...

The atria, the upper chambers, are separated by the interatrial septum. They receive blood returning to the heart and pump blood into the ventricles.

...where the blood comes in

The right atrium receives blood from the superior and inferior venae cavae. The left atrium, which is smaller but has thicker walls than the right atrium, forms the uppermost part of the heart's left border. It receives blood from the two pulmonary veins.

Downstairs...

The right and left ventricles, which are separated by the interventricular septum, make up the two lower chambers. The ventricles receive blood from the atria. Composed of highly developed musculature, the ventricles are larger and have thicker walls than the atria.

...where the blood goes out

The right ventricle receives blood from the right atrium and pumps it through the pulmonary arteries to the lungs. The left ventricle, which is larger than the right, receives oxygenated blood from the left atrium and pumps it through the aorta to all other vessels of the body.

> The heart valves prevent deoxygenated blood from mixing with oxygenated blood, so that the body always gets the proper "fuel."

The valves

The heart contains four valves, two AV valves and two semilunar valves.

Valve job

The valves allow forward flow of blood through the heart and prevent backward flow. They open and close in response to

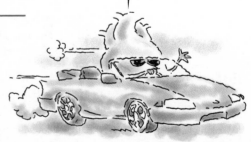

pressure changes caused by ventricular contraction and blood ejection.

The two AV valves separate the atria from the ventricles. The right AV valve, called the *tricuspid valve*, prevents backflow from the right ventricle into the right atrium. The left AV valve, called the *mitral valve*, prevents backflow from the left ventricle into the left atrium.

One of the two semilunar valves is the *pulmonic valve*, which prevents backflow from the pulmonary artery into the right ventricle. The other semilunar valve is the *aortic valve*, which prevents backflow from the aorta into the left ventricle.

Counting cusps

The tricuspid valve has three triangular cusps, or leaflets. The mitral valve, also called the *bicuspid valve*, contains two cusps, a large anterior and a smaller posterior. Chordae tendineae (tendinous cords) attach the cusps of the two AV valves to papillary muscles in the ventricles. These cords vary in length and thickness and, in many cases, branch out. The semilunar valves have three cusps that are shaped like half-moons—hence, the name *semilunar*.

Memory jogger

If you can remember that there are two sets of heart valves, you can recall that there are two distinct heart sounds. Closure of the atrioventricular valves makes the first heart sound, the *lub*; closure of the semilunar valves makes the second heart sound, the *dub*.

Heart function

The heart's job is to keep blood flowing throughout the circulatory system, delivering oxygen and removing waste products from the body's cells. The heart actually consists of two separate pumps, one on the right and one on the left.

Exit stage left

Specifically, the left side of the heart pumps out oxygenated blood, which the circulatory system delivers to all the body's tissues. The cells take up the oxygen and release carbon dioxide, a waste product. The circulatory system then carries the deoxygenated blood back to the right side of the heart.

Enter stage right

After receiving blood from the systemic circulation, the right side of the heart pumps it to the lungs. There, the blood releases carbon dioxide, which the lungs excrete. The blood also picks up oxygen from the lungs. The oxy-

Pathways of oxygenated and deoxygenated blood

Oxygenated blood travels from the lungs to the left side of the heart, where it's pumped out to the body. Deoxygenated blood returns to the right side of the heart, where it's pumped back to the lungs.

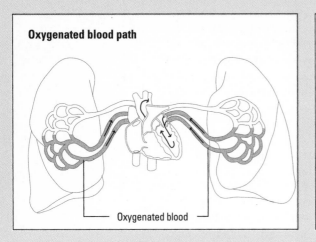

Oxygenated blood path

Oxygenated blood

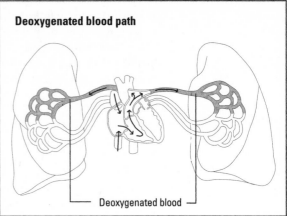

Deoxygenated blood path

Deoxygenated blood

genated blood then travels back to the left side of the heart, where the process begins again. (See *Pathways of oxygenated and deoxygenated blood.*)

Workaholic

The average healthy adult heart pumps approximately 5 to 7 L of blood per minute, or 1,500 to 2,000 gallons per day. The heart performs this task continuously throughout a person's life; however, pumping efficiency can change with age. (See *Cardiovascular changes with aging.*)

Heart conduction

The heart's conduction system consists of specialized cells and fibers that produce electrical impulses. These electrical impulses discharge automatically, causing the heart muscles to contract and pump blood through the body. The heart's pattern of contraction and relaxation is called the *cardiac cycle.* (See *Cardiac conduction system*, page 8.)

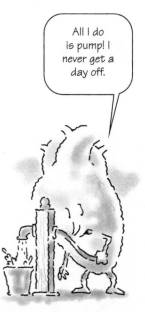

All I do is pump! I never get a day off.

Ages and stages

Cardiovascular changes with aging

As a normal part of aging, contractile strength declines, making the heart less efficient. In most people, resting cardiac output diminishes 30% to 35% by age 70.

In addition, veins dilate and stretch with age, and coronary artery blood flow drops 35% between ages 20 and 60. The aorta becomes more rigid, causing systolic blood pressure to rise disproportionately higher than diastolic pressure, resulting in a widened pulse pressure.

Between ages 30 and 80, the left ventricular wall grows 25% thicker from its increased efforts to pump blood. Heart valves also become thicker from fibrotic and sclerotic changes. This thickening can prevent the valves from closing completely, causing systolic murmurs.

Electrical impulses

The conduction system of the heart contains pacemaker cells that have three unique characteristics:
• automaticity — the ability to generate an electrical impulse automatically
• conductivity — the ability to pass the impulse to the next cell
• contractility — the ability to shorten the fibers in the heart when receiving the impulse.

Setting the pace

The sinoatrial (SA) node — located on the endocardial surface of the right atrium, just below the entrance of the superior vena cava — is the normal pacemaker of the heart. As such, it generates electrical impulses between 60 and 100 times per minute. The firing of the SA node spreads each impulse throughout the right and left atria, resulting in atrial contraction.

Cardiac conduction system

Specialized fibers propagate electrical impulses throughout the heart's cells, causing the heart to contract. This illustration shows the elements of the cardiac conduction system.

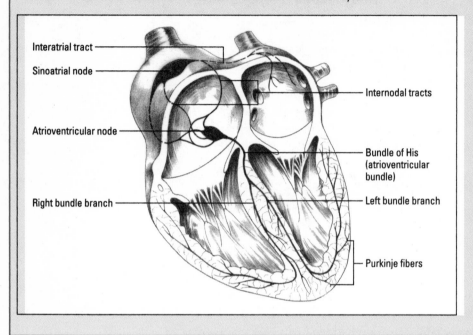

Interatrial tract

Sinoatrial node

Atrioventricular node

Right bundle branch

Internodal tracts

Bundle of His (atrioventricular bundle)

Left bundle branch

Purkinje fibers

Waiting for results

The AV node, situated low in the septal wall of the right atrium, receives the impulse from the SA node and slows impulse conduction between the atria and ventricles. This "resistor" node allows time for the contracting atria to fill the ventricles with blood before the lower chambers contract.

Shock wave

From the AV node, the impulse travels to the bundle of His (modified cardiac muscle fibers), branching off to the right and left bundles. Finally, the impulse travels to tiny Purkinje fibers, the distal portions of the left and right bundle branches. These fibers fan across the surface of the ventricles from the endocardium to the myocardium. As the impulse spreads, it brings word to the blood-filled ventricles to contract.

Backup plan

The conduction system has two built-in safety mechanisms. If the SA node fails to fire, the AV node generates impulses between 40 and 60 times per minute. If the SA node and the AV node fail, the ventricles can generate their own impulses between 20 and 40 times per minute.

> A precise series of electrical and mechanical events must occur before each heart beat. That's an engineering phenomenon!

Cardiac cycle

The cardiac cycle is the period from the beginning of one heartbeat to the beginning of the next. During this cycle, electrical and mechanical events must occur in the proper sequence and to the proper degree to provide adequate blood flow to all body parts. The cardiac cycle has two phases: systole (contraction) and diastole (relaxation). (See *Events in the cardiac cycle*, page 10.)

Contract...

At the beginning of atrial systole, the atria, which are filled with blood, contract and push blood into the ventricles. After the ventricles fill, ventricular systole occurs and the ventricles contract. Ventricular blood pressure builds until it exceeds the pressures in the pulmonary artery and the aorta. The pressure creates enough force to close the AV valves (mitral and tricuspid) and to open the semilunar valves (pulmonic and aortic). When the semilunar valves open, the ventricles eject blood into the aorta and the pulmonary artery.

...and release

When the ventricles empty and relax, ventricular pressure falls below the pressures in the pulmonary artery and the aorta. At the beginning of diastole, the semilunar valves close to prevent the backflow of blood into the ventricles, and the mitral and tricuspid valves open, allowing blood to flow into the ventricles from the atria.

When the ventricles become full, near the end of this phase, the atria contract to send the remaining blood to the ventricles. Then a new cardiac cycle begins as the heart enters systole again.

The specs for this cycle's engine

Cardiac output (CO) refers to the amount of blood the heart pumps in 1 minute. It's equal to the heart rate (HR)

Events in the cardiac cycle

The cardiac cycle consists of five events, as described here.

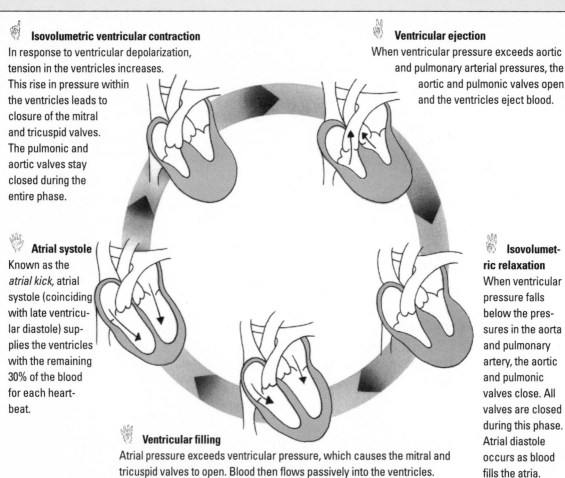

Isovolumetric ventricular contraction
In response to ventricular depolarization, tension in the ventricles increases. This rise in pressure within the ventricles leads to closure of the mitral and tricuspid valves. The pulmonic and aortic valves stay closed during the entire phase.

Ventricular ejection
When ventricular pressure exceeds aortic and pulmonary arterial pressures, the aortic and pulmonic valves open and the ventricles eject blood.

Atrial systole
Known as the *atrial kick,* atrial systole (coinciding with late ventricular diastole) supplies the ventricles with the remaining 30% of the blood for each heartbeat.

Isovolumetric relaxation
When ventricular pressure falls below the pressures in the aorta and pulmonary artery, the aortic and pulmonic valves close. All valves are closed during this phase. Atrial diastole occurs as blood fills the atria.

Ventricular filling
Atrial pressure exceeds ventricular pressure, which causes the mitral and tricuspid valves to open. Blood then flows passively into the ventricles. About 70% of ventricular filling takes place during this phase.

multiplied by the stroke volume (SV), the amount of blood ejected with each heartbeat (CO = HR × SV). Stroke volume, in turn, depends on three major factors: preload, contractility, and afterload. To determine SV, use the equation SV = CO ÷ HR. (See *Understanding preload, contractility, and afterload.*)

Understanding preload, contractility, and afterload

Thinking of the heart as a balloon can help you understand the three factors that determine stroke volume.

Blowing up the balloon

Preload is the stretching of muscle fibers in the ventricles. This stretching results from blood volume in the ventricles at end-diastole. According to *Starling's law,* the more the heart muscles stretch during diastole, the more forcefully they contract during systole. Think of preload as the balloon stretching as air is blown into it. The more air, the greater the stretch.

The balloon's stretch

Contractility refers to the inherent ability of the myocardium to contract normally. Contractility is influenced by preload. The greater the stretch, the more forceful the contraction—or, the more air in the balloon, the greater the stretch, and the farther the balloon will fly when air is allowed to expel.

The knot that ties the balloon

Afterload refers to the pressure that the ventricular muscles must generate to overcome the higher pressure in the aorta to get the blood out of the heart. *Resistance* is the knot on the end of the balloon, which the balloon has to work against to get the air out.

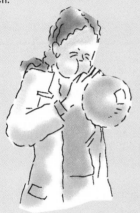
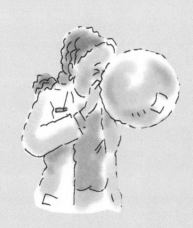
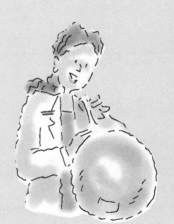

Vascular system

As blood makes its way through the vascular system, it travels through five distinct types of blood vessels, involving three methods of circulation.

Blood vessels

The five types of blood vessels are:

 arteries

 arterioles

veins

 venules

capillaries.

The structure of each type of vessel differs according to its function in the cardiovascular system and the pressure exerted by the volume of blood at various sites within the system.

Outbound

Arteries and arterioles carry blood away from the heart. Nearly all arteries carry oxygen-rich blood from the heart throughout the rest of the body. The only exception is the pulmonary artery, which carries oxygen-depleted blood from the right ventricle to the lungs.

Through thick...

Arteries have thick, muscular walls to accommodate the flow of blood at high speeds and pressures. These walls contain a tough, elastic layer that helps propel blood through the arterial system.

Arterioles have thinner walls than arteries. They constrict or dilate to control blood flow to the capillaries.

...and thin

Vein walls are thinner than artery walls because of the low blood pressures of venous return to the heart. Veins also have larger diameters and are more pliable than arteries. That pliablility allows veins to accommodate variations in blood volume.

Venules gather blood from the capillaries; their walls are thinner than those of arterioles.

Inbound

Veins and venules carry blood toward the heart. Nearly all veins carry oxygen-depleted blood. The only exception is the pulmonary vein, which carries oxygenated blood from the lungs to the left atrium. Veins serve as a large reservoir for circulating blood. They contain valves at periodic intervals to prevent blood from flowing backward.

Capital capillaries

The exchange of fluid, nutrients, and metabolic wastes between blood and cells occurs in the capillaries. This exchange can occur because capillaries are thin-walled (they're composed of only a single layer of epithelial cells) and highly permeable. About 5% of circulating blood volume at any given moment is contained within the capillary network. Capillaries are connected to the arteries and veins through the arterioles and venules, respectively.

Free to roam

About 60,000 miles of arteries, arterioles, capillaries, venules, and veins keep blood circulating to and from every functioning cell in the body. (See *Major blood vessels*, page 14.)

Circulation

Three methods of circulation carry blood throughout the body: pulmonary, systemic, and coronary.

Pulmonary circulation

In pulmonary circulation, blood travels to the lungs to pick up oxygen and release carbon dioxide.

Returns and exchanges

As the blood moves from the heart to the lungs and back again, it proceeds as follows:
• Deoxygenated blood travels from the right ventricle through the pulmonic valve into the pulmonary arteries.
• Blood passes through progressively smaller arteries and arterioles into the capillaries of the lungs.
• Blood reaches the alveoli and exchanges carbon dioxide for oxygen.
• Oxygenated blood then returns via venules and veins to the pulmonary veins, which carry it back to the heart's left atrium.

Systemic circulation

Systemic circulation begins when blood pumped from the left ventricle carries oxygen and other nutrients to body cells. This same circulation also transports waste products for excretion.

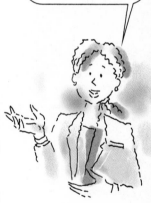

The circulatory system is amazing! Blood travels through three circulatory paths just to keep the body functioning.

Major blood vessels

This illustration shows the body's major arteries and veins.

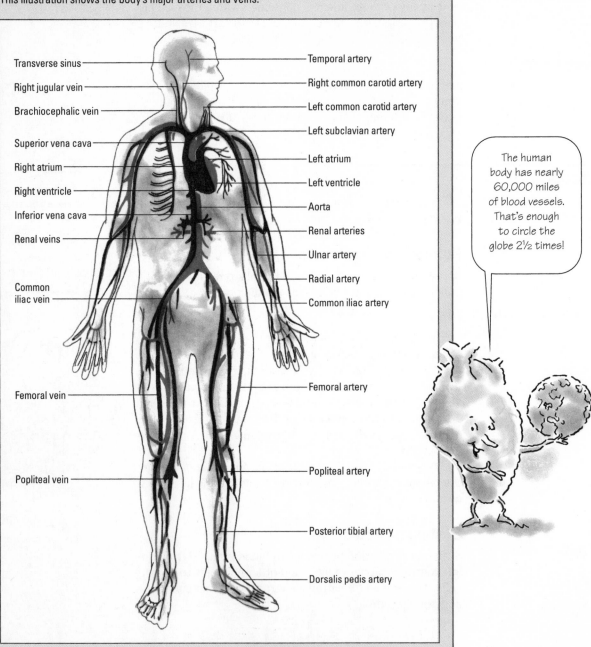

The human body has nearly 60,000 miles of blood vessels. That's enough to circle the globe 2½ times!

Supply routes

The major artery, the aorta, branches into vessels that supply specific organs and areas of the body. As it arches out of the top of the heart and down to the abdomen, three arteries branch off the top of the arch to supply the upper body with blood:
• The left common carotid artery supplies blood to the brain.
• The left subclavian artery supplies blood to the arms.
• The innominate artery supplies blood to the upper chest.
   As the aorta descends through the thorax and abdomen, its branches supply the organs of the GI and genitourinary systems, spinal column, and lower chest and abdominal muscles. Then the aorta divides into the iliac arteries, which further divide into femoral arteries.

Divide and conquer

As the arteries divide into smaller units, the number of vessels increases dramatically, thereby increasing the area of tissue to which blood flows, also called the *area of perfusion*.

Dilation is another part of the equation

At the end of the arterioles and the beginning of the capillaries, strong sphincters control blood flow into the tissues. These sphincters dilate to permit more flow when needed, close to shunt blood to other areas, or constrict to increase blood pressure.

A large area of low pressure

Although the capillary bed contains the smallest vessels, it supplies blood to the largest number of cells. Capillary pressure is extremely low to allow for the exchange of nutrients, oxygen, and carbon dioxide with body cells. From the capillaries, blood flows into the venules and, eventually, into the veins.

Upward mobility

Valves in the veins prevent blood backflow. Pooled blood in each valved segment travels toward the heart by pressure from the moving volume of blood from below.
   The veins merge until they form two main branches, the superior vena cava and inferior vena cava, which return blood to the right atrium.

Coronary circulation

The heart relies on the coronary arteries and their branches for its supply of oxygenated blood. It depends on the cardiac veins to remove oxygen-depleted blood. (See *Vessels that supply the heart*.)

The heart gets its part

During left ventricular systole, blood is ejected into the aorta. During diastole, blood flows out of the heart and then through the coronary arteries to nourish the heart muscle.

From the right...

The right coronary artery supplies blood to the right atrium, part of the left atrium, most of the right ventricle, and the inferior part of the left ventricle.

Vessels that supply the heart

Coronary circulation involves the arterial system of blood vessels that supply oxygenated blood to the heart and the venous system that removes oxygen-depleted blood from it.

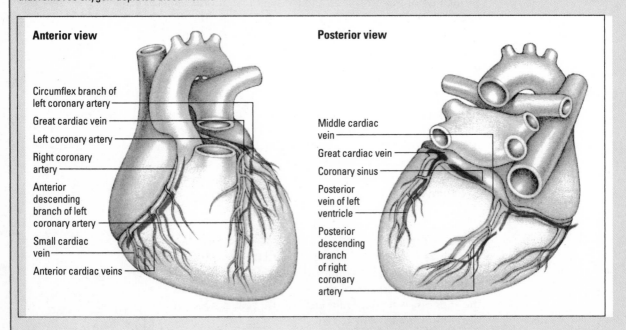

Anterior view

Circumflex branch of left coronary artery
Great cardiac vein
Left coronary artery
Right coronary artery
Anterior descending branch of left coronary artery
Small cardiac vein
Anterior cardiac veins

Posterior view

Middle cardiac vein
Great cardiac vein
Coronary sinus
Posterior vein of left ventricle
Posterior descending branch of right coronary artery

...and from the left

The left coronary artery, which splits into the anterior descending artery and circumflex artery, supplies blood to the left atrium, most of the left ventricle, and most of the interventricular septum.

Superficially speaking

The cardiac veins lie superficial to the arteries. The largest vein, the coronary sinus, opens into the right atrium. Most of the major cardiac veins empty into the coronary sinus, except for the anterior cardiac veins, which empty into the right atrium.

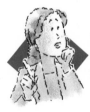

Quick quiz

1. The ventricles receive blood from the:
   A. superior vena cava.
   B. inferior vena cava.
   C. pulmonary veins.
   D. atria.

Answer: D. The ventricles receive blood from the atria. The atria receive blood returning from the body. Specifically, the superior and inferior venae cavae supply blood to the right atrium and the pulmonic veins supply blood to the left atria.

2. To control blood flow through the heart, the heart has:
   A. two valves.
   B. four valves.
   C. six valves.
   D. eight valves.

Answer: B. The heart has two AV valves (the tricuspid and mitral valves) that prevent the backflow of blood from the ventricles to the atria and two semilunar valves (the pulmonic and aortic valves) that prevent the backflow of blood from the arteries to the ventricles.

3. The normal pacemaker of the heart is the:
   A. SA node.
   B. AV node.
   C. ventricles.
   D. Purkinje fibers.

Answer: A. The SA node is the normal pacemaker of the heart, generating impulses 60 to 100 times per minute. The AV node is the secondary pacemaker of the heart (generating 40 to 60 beats per minute). The ventricles are the last line of defense (generating 20 to 40 beats per minute).

4. Which of the following options isn't one of the three methods of circulation?
    A.   Pulmonary circulation
    B.   Aortic circulation
    C.   Coronary circulation
    D.   Systemic circulation

Answer: B. The three methods of circulation are pulmonary circulation, which carries blood to and from the lungs; systemic circulation, which carries blood to and from the body; and coronary circulation, which carries blood to and from the heart.

5. Cardiac output (the amount of blood the heart pumps in 1 minute) is equal to:
    A.   preload plus afterload.
    B.   stroke volume.
    C.   heart rate.
    D.   heart rate multiplied by stroke volume.

Answer: D. Cardiac output is equal to the heart rate multiplied by stroke volume (the amount of blood ejected with each heartbeat).

Scoring

☆☆☆   If you answered all five questions correctly, marvelous! You've gotten to the heart of cardiovascular anatomy and physiology.

☆☆   If you answered four questions correctly, great! We won't call you "vein" if you're a little proud of yourself.

☆   If you answered fewer than four questions correctly, take heart! Circulate through this chapter again and you're sure to do better.

2

Assessment

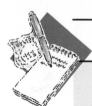

Just the facts

In this chapter, you'll learn:

♦ methods for obtaining a health history

♦ techniques for assessing the heart and vascular system

♦ normal and abnormal assessment findings.

A look at cardiovascular assessment

Performed correctly, cardiovascular assessment can help to identify and evaluate changes in the patient's cardiac function. Baseline information obtained during assessment helps guide diagnosis, intervention, and follow-up care. Complete cardiovascular assessment of a patient consists of obtaining an accurate, thorough health history and performing a physical examination, including assessing the patient's heart and vascular system.

Note, however, if your patient is in a cardiac crisis, you'll have to rethink your assessment priorities. The patient's condition and the clinical situation dictate what steps you should take.

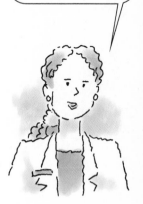

Base your assessment priorities on the patient's physical condition. If he's in a cardiac crisis, focus your care on his immediate needs.

Obtaining a health history

Begin your cardiovascular assessment by introducing yourself to the patient and explaining what will occur during the health history and physical examination. For the history portion of your assessment, ask about the patient's chief complaint as well as personal and family history of disease. Be sure to document all of your findings.

Key questions for assessing cardiac function

The following questions and statements will help you to assess the patient more accurately:
- Tell me about any feelings of shortness of breath you have. Does a particular body position seem to bring this on? Which one? How long does shortness of breath last? What relieves it?
- Has sudden breathing trouble ever awakened you from sleep? Tell me more about this.
- Do you use more than one pillow at night to help you breathe? If so, how many?
- Do you ever wake up coughing? How often? Have you ever coughed up blood?

- Does your heart ever pound, beat fast, flutter, or skip a beat? If so, when does this happen?
- Do you ever get dizzy or faint? What seems to bring this on?
- Tell me about any swelling in your hands, ankles, or feet. What time of day does this usually occur? Does anything relieve the swelling?
- Have you noticed any changes in color, temperature, or sensation in your legs? If so, which leg? Describe the changes.
- Do you urinate frequently at night?
- Tell me how you feel while you're doing your daily activities. Have you had to limit your activities or rest often while doing them?

Chief complaint

Begin the health history by asking the patient why he's seeking medical care. If he has chest pain, ask him to rate the pain on a scale of 1 to 10, in which 1 means that the pain is negligible and 10 means it's the worst pain imaginable. Ask about the location, radiation, and duration of pain and any precipitating, exacerbating, or relieving factors. Also ask the patient if he has experienced any other symptoms, such as dizziness, nausea, or sweating.

Let the patient describe his problem in his own words. Avoid leading questions. If the patient isn't in distress, ask questions requiring more than a "yes" or "no" response. (See *Key questions for assessing cardiac function*.)

Other ailments

Patients with cardiovascular problems also frequently complain of headaches, shortness of breath, dizziness, excess fatigue, unexplained weight changes, high or low blood pressure, pain in the extremities (such as leg pain or cramps), and swelling of the extremities. (See *Pregnancy and vein changes*.) They may also report peripheral skin changes, such as decreased hair distribution, skin color changes, or a thin, shiny appearance of the skin.

Pregnancy and vein changes

You might find 4+ pitting edema in the legs of a pregnant patient in her third trimester. Severe edema is common not just in the third trimester but also in pregnant women who stand for long periods. Varicose veins are another common finding in the third trimester.

Ages and stages

At risk for cardiovascular disease

As you analyze a patient's problems, remember that age, sex, and race are essential considerations in identifying patients at risk for cardiovascular disorders. For example, coronary artery disease most commonly affects white men between ages 40 and 60. Hypertension occurs most often in blacks.

Women are also vulnerable to heart disease, especially postmenopausal women and those with diabetes mellitus. Many elderly people have increased systolic blood pressure because of an increase in the rigidity of their blood vessel walls with age. Overall, elderly people have a higher incidence of cardiovascular disease than do younger people.

Personal and family history

After you've asked about the patient's chief complaint, inquire about his personal and family medical history, including heart disease, diabetes, or chronic lung, kidney, or liver disease. (See *At risk for cardiovascular disease*.)

Also ask the patient about his:
• stress level and coping mechanisms
• current health habits, such as smoking, alcohol intake, caffeine intake, exercise, and dietary intake of fat and sodium
• drug use, including over-the-counter drugs, vitamins, and herbal preparations
• previous operations
• environmental or occupational hazards
• activities of daily living.

Performing a physical assessment

Cardiovascular disease affects people of all ages and can take many forms. A consistent, methodical approach to assessment can help you identify abnormalities. As always, the key to accurate assessment is regular practice, which helps to improve technique and efficiency.

Before you begin your physical assessment, you'll need a stethoscope with a bell and a diaphragm, an appropriate-sized blood pressure cuff, a ruler, and a penlight or other flexible light source. Also, make sure the room is quiet.

Ask the patient to remove all clothing except his underwear and to put on an examination gown. Have the patient lie on his back, with the head of the examination table at a 30- to 45-degree angle, depending on the patient's comfort level and respiratory status. Stand on the patient's right side if you're right-handed or his left side if you're left-handed so you can auscultate more easily.

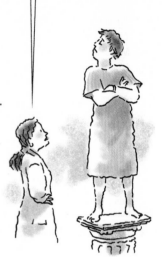

I'm sorry, but I can't assess you from there. You'll need to lie down on the examination table.

Assessing the heart

Assessing the heart involves inspection, palpation, percussion, and auscultation.

Inspection

First, take a moment to assess the patient's general appearance. Is he overly thin? Obese? Alert? Anxious? Next, inspect the patient's precordium (the anterior region of the chest and thorax, including the epigastric area). Note landmarks you can use to describe your findings as well as structures underlying the chest wall. (See *Inspecting and palpating the precordium.*)

Heave, ho!

Also look for pulsations, symmetry of movement, retractions, or heaves. A heave is a strong outward thrust of the chest wall that occurs during systole. Note any deviations from the typical chest shape and movement.

Shed some light on the matter

Position a light source, such as a flashlight or gooseneck lamp, so that it casts a shadow on the patient's chest. Note the location of the apical pulse. Located in the fifth intercostal space medial to the left midclavicular line, the apical pulse is usually the point of maximal impulse. Because it corresponds to the apex of the heart, the apical pulse indicates how well the left ventricle is working.

The apical pulse can be seen in about 50% of adults. You'll notice it more easily in children and in patients with thin chest walls. For obese patients or patients with large breasts, ask them to sit up and lean forward during in-

Memory jogger

To remember the order in which you should perform assessment of the cardiovascular system, just think, "I'll Properly Perform Assessment."

Inspection

Palpation

Percussion

Auscultation

Inspecting and palpating the precordium

Use the following guidelines when inspecting and palpating the precordium:
• Locate the six precordial areas by using the anatomic landmarks named for the underlying structures.
• Palpate (or inspect) the *sternoclavicular area,* which lies at the top of the sternum at the junction of the clavicles.
• Move to the *aortic area,* located in the second intercostal space on the right sternal border.
• Assess the *pulmonary area,* found in the second intercostal space on the left sternal border.

• Palpate the *right ventricular area* (the point where the fifth rib joins the left sternal border).
• Then assess the *left ventricular area (apical area),* which falls at the fifth intercostal space at the midclavicular line.
• Finally, palpate the *epigastric area* at the base of the sternum between the cartilage of the left and right seventh ribs. Avoid pressing on the xiphoid process.
    The views below show where to find critical landmarks used in cardiovascular assessment.

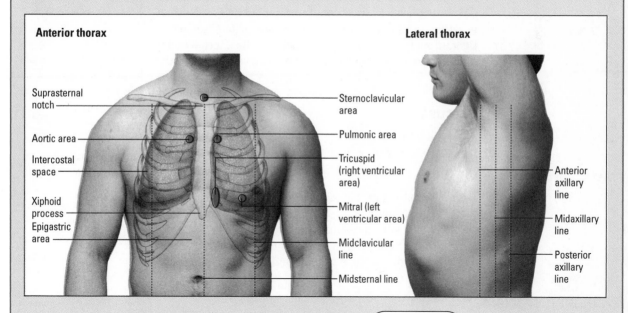

Anterior thorax

Suprasternal notch

Aortic area

Intercostal space

Xiphoid process

Epigastric area

Sternoclavicular area

Pulmonic area

Tricuspid (right ventricular area)

Mitral (left ventricular area)

Midclavicular line

Midsternal line

Lateral thorax

Anterior axillary line

Midaxillary line

Posterior axillary line

spection. This brings the heart closer to the anterior chest wall and makes pulsations more noticeable. To find the apical pulse in a woman with large breasts, displace the breasts during the examination.

Palpation

Maintain a gentle touch when you palpate so that you won't obscure pulsations or similar findings. Using the ball of

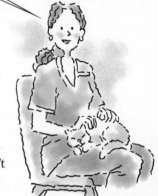

Use a gentle touch when you palpate. Some findings will be as subtle as a cat's purr.

your hand, then your fingertips, palpate over the precordium to find the apical pulse. Note heaves or thrills, fine vibrations that feel like the purring of a cat. (See *Assessing the apical pulse*.)

The apical pulse may be difficult to palpate in obese and pregnant patients and in patients with thick chest walls. If it's difficult to palpate with the patient lying on his back, have him lie on his left side or sit upright. It may also be helpful to have the patient exhale completely and hold his breath for a few seconds.

Pulseless

Also palpate the sternoclavicular, aortic, pulmonic, tricuspid, and epigastric areas for abnormal pulsations. Normally, you won't feel pulsations in those areas. In a thin patient, though, an aortic arch pulsation in the sternoclavicular area or an abdominal aorta pulsation in the epigastric area may be a normal finding.

Percussion

Although percussion isn't as useful as other methods of cardiac assessment, it may help you locate cardiac borders.

Border patrol

Begin percussing at the anterior axillary line and continue toward the sternum along the fifth intercostal space. The sound changes from resonance to dullness over the left border of the heart, normally at the midclavicular line. The right border of the heart is usually aligned with the sternum and can't be percussed.

Percussion problems

Percussion may be difficult in obese patients (because of the fat overlying the chest) or in female patients (because of breast tissue). In this case, a chest X-ray can provide more accurate information about the heart border.

Auscultation

You can learn a great deal about the heart by auscultating for heart sounds. Cardiac auscultation requires a methodical approach and lots of practice. Begin by warming the stethoscope in your hands and then identify the sites where you'll auscultate: over the four cardiac valves and at Erb's point, the third intercostal space at the left sternal border.

Assessing the apical pulse

The apical pulse is associated with the first heart sound and carotid pulsation. To ensure that you're feeling the apical pulse and not a muscle spasm or some other pulsation, use one hand to palpate the patient's carotid artery and the other to palpate the apical pulse. Then compare the timing and regularity of the impulses. The apical pulse should roughly coincide with the carotid pulsation.

Note the amplitude, size, intensity, location, and duration of the apical pulse. You should feel a gentle pulsation in an area about ½″ to ¾″ (1.5 to 2 cm) in diameter.

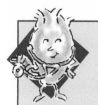

Location, location, location

Sites for heart sounds

When auscultating for heart sounds, place the stethoscope over the four different sites illustrated at right.

Normal heart sounds indicate events in the cardiac cycle, such as the closing of heart valves, and are reflected to specific areas of the chest wall. Auscultation sites are identified by the names of heart valves but aren't located directly over the valves. Rather, these sites are located along the pathway blood takes as it flows through the heart's chambers and valves.

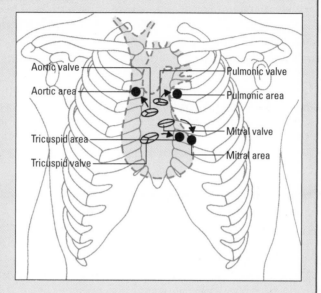

Use the bell to hear low-pitched sounds and the diaphragm to hear high-pitched sounds. (See *Sites for heart sounds.*)

A sound process

Auscultate for heart sounds with the patient in three positions: lying on his back with the head of the bed raised 30 to 45 degrees, sitting up, and lying on his left side. Use a zigzag pattern over the precordium. You can start at the apex and work downward or at the base and work upward. Whichever approach you use, be consistent.

Use the diaphragm to listen as you go in one direction; use the bell as you come back in the other direction. Be sure to listen over the entire precordium, not just over the valves.

Note the heart rate and rhythm. Always identify the first and second heart sounds, and then listen for adventitious sounds, such as third and fourth heart sounds, murmurs, and rubs. (For more information on auscultating heart sounds, see chapter 3, Cardiac auscultation.)

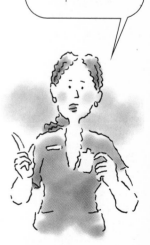

Be sure to be consistent in the way you perform auscultation of the pericardium.

Assessing the vascular system

Assessment of the vascular system is an important part of a full cardiovascular assessment. Your vascular assessment begins with assessing the vital signs, including the patient's temperature, blood pressure, pulse rate, and respiratory rate. In addition, measure the patient's height and weight because these measurements help determine cardiovascular risk factors, determine medication dosages, and detect fluid overload. Then proceed with your examination. Examination of the patient's arms and legs can reveal arterial or venous disorders. Examine the arms when you take vital signs. Check the legs later during the physical examination, when the patient is lying on his back. Remember to evaluate leg veins when the patient is standing.

A thorough inspection should be the first step in any assessment.

Inspection

Start your assessment of the vascular system the same way you start an assessment of the cardiac system—by making general observations. Are the arms equal in size? Are the legs symmetrical?

Inspect the skin. It should be warm. Note the color of the skin. Also note how body hair is distributed. Hair should be distributed symmetrically. Note lesions, scars, clubbing, and edema of the extremities. If the patient is confined to bed, check the sacrum for swelling. Examine the fingernails; they should be pink, firm, and free from markings.

Moving in for a closer look

Next, move on to a closer inspection. Start by observing the vessels in the patient's neck. Inspection of these vessels can provide information about blood volume and pressure in the right side of the heart. The carotid artery should appear to have a brisk, localized pulsation. This pulsation doesn't decrease when the patient is upright, when he inhales, or when you palpate the carotid. Note whether the pulsations are weak or bounding.

Inspect the jugular veins. The internal jugular vein has a softer, undulating pulsation. Unlike the pulsation of the carotid artery, pulsation of the internal jugular vein changes in response to position, breathing, and palpation. The vein normally protrudes when the patient is lying down and lies flat when he stands.

Take this lying down

To check the jugular venous pulse, have the patient lie on his back. Elevate the head of the bed 30 to 45 degrees and turn the patient's head slightly away from you. Normally, the highest pulsation occurs no more than 1½″ (4 cm) above the sternal notch. Pulsations above that point indicate an elevation in central venous pressure and jugular vein distention.

Palpation

The first step in palpation is to assess the patient's skin temperature, texture, and turgor. Then check capillary refill by assessing the nail beds on the fingers and toes. Refill time should be no more than 3 seconds, or the time it takes to say "capillary refill."

Palpate the patient's arms and legs for temperature and edema. Edema is graded on a four-point scale. If your finger leaves a slight imprint, the edema is recorded as +1. If your finger leaves a deep imprint that slowly returns to normal, the edema is recorded as +4.

Top down

Also palpate for arterial pulses. (Arterial pulses are pressure waves of blood generated by the pumping action of the heart. All vessels in the arterial system have pulsations, but pulsations can be felt only where an artery lies near the skin.)

Palpate for arterial pulses by gently pressing with the pads of your index and middle fingers. Start at the top of the patient's body at the temporal artery and work your way down. Check the carotid, brachial, radial, femoral, popliteal, posterior tibial, and dorsalis pedis pulses on each side of the body, comparing pulse volume and symmetry. *Don't palpate both carotid arteries at the same time or press too firmly. If you do, the patient may faint or become bradycardic.* If you haven't put on gloves for the examination, do so when you palpate the femoral arteries.

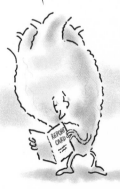

Gee... I feel like I'm pumping hard enough, but my pulses received a poor grade for strength.

Making the grade

All pulses should be regular in rhythm and equal in strength. Pulses are graded on the following scale: 4+ is bounding, 3+ is increased, 2+ is normal, 1+ is weak, and 0 is absent. (See *Assessing arterial pulses*, page 28.)

Assessing arterial pulses

To assess arterial pulses, apply pressure with your index and middle fingers. The following illustrations show where to position your fingers when palpating for various pulses.

Carotid pulse
Lightly place your fingers just medial to the trachea and below the jaw angle. Never palpate both carotid arteries at the same time.

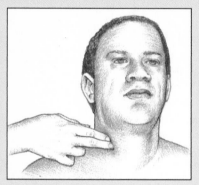

Brachial pulse
Position your fingers medial to the biceps tendon.

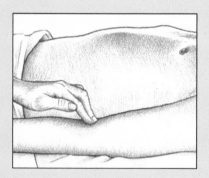

Radial pulse
Apply gentle pressure to the medial and ventral side of the wrist, just below the base of the thumb.

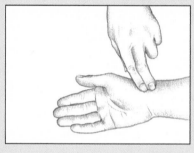

Femoral pulse
Press relatively hard at a point inferior to the inguinal ligament. For an obese patient, palpate in the crease of the groin, halfway between the pubic bone and hip bone.

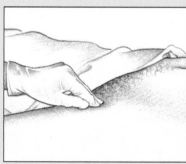

Popliteal pulse
Press firmly in the popliteal fossa at the back of the knee.

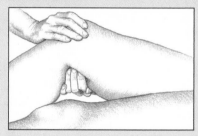

Posterior tibial pulse
Apply pressure behind and slightly below the malleolus of the ankle.

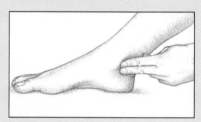

Dorsalis pedis pulse
Place your fingers on the medial dorsum of the foot while the patient points his toes down. The pulse is difficult to palpate here and may seem to be absent in healthy patients.

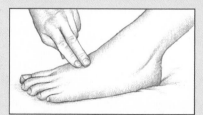

Now hear this!

Performing arterial auscultation

Use these steps when auscultating the carotid, femoral, and popliteal arteries and the abdominal aorta:

• Ask the patient to hold his breath while you auscultate.

• Assess the carotid arteries by auscultating with the bell of the stethoscope on both sides of the trachea, as shown at right.

• To evaluate the femoral and popliteal arteries, place the bell of the stethoscope over the pulse sites that you palpated earlier in the assessment.

• Auscultate the abdominal aorta by listening to the epigastric area.

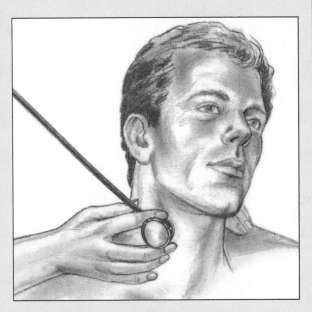

Auscultation

After you palpate, use the bell of the stethoscope to begin auscultation. Following the palpation sequence, listen over each artery. You shouldn't hear sounds over the carotid arteries. A hum, also called a *bruit*, sounds like buzzing or blowing and could indicate arteriosclerotic plaque formation. (See *Performing arterial auscultation.*)

Assess the upper abdomen for abnormal pulsations, which could indicate the presence of an abdominal aortic aneurysm. Finally, auscultate the femoral and popliteal pulses, checking for a bruit or other abnormal sounds.

Interpreting abnormal findings

This section outlines some common abnormal cardiovascular system assessment findings and their causes.

Abnormal skin and hair findings

Cyanosis, pallor, and cool or cold skin may indicate poor cardiac output and tissue perfusion. Conditions causing fever or increased cardiac output may make the skin feel warmer than normal. Absence of body hair on the arms or legs may indicate diminished arterial blood flow to those areas. Spongy fingernails indicate clubbing, a sign of chronic hypoxia. Red or brown splinter lines on fingernails suggest bacterial endocarditis.

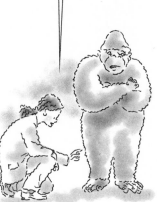

Hmmm. No absence of body hair here.

How swell!

Swelling, or edema, may indicate heart failure or venous insufficiency. It may also be caused by varicosities or thrombophlebitis.

Chronic right-sided heart failure may cause ascites and generalized edema. If the patient has compression of a vein in a specific area, he may have localized swelling along the path of the compressed vessel. Right-sided heart failure may cause swelling in the lower legs. (See *Findings in arterial and venous insufficiency*.)

Abnormal pulsations

A displaced apical impulse may indicate an enlarged left ventricle, which can result from heart failure or hypertension. A forceful apical impulse, or one lasting longer than one-third of the cardiac cycle, may point to increased cardiac output. If you find a pulsation in the patient's aortic, pulmonic, or tricuspid area, his heart chamber may be enlarged or he may have valvular disease.

Unpredictable pulses

Increased cardiac output or an aortic aneurysm may also produce pulsations in the aortic area. A patient with an epigastric pulsation may have early heart failure or an aortic aneurysm. A pulsation in the sternoclavicular area suggests an aortic aneurysm. A patient with anemia, anxiety, increased cardiac output, or a thin chest wall might have slight pulsations to the right and left of the sternum.

Weak vs. strong

A weak arterial pulse may indicate decreased cardiac output or increased peripheral vascular resistance, both of which point to arterial atherosclerotic disease. Many elderly patients have weak pedal pulses.

Findings in arterial and venous insufficiency

Assessment findings in patients with arterial insufficiency differ from those associated with chronic venous insufficiency. These illustrations show those differences.

Arterial insufficiency
In a patient with arterial insufficiency, pulses may be decreased or absent. His skin will be cool, pale, and shiny, and he may have pain in his legs and feet. Ulcerations typically occur in the area around the toes, and the foot usually turns deep red when dependent. Nails may be thick and ridged.

Chronic venous insufficiency
In a patient with chronic venous insufficiency, check for ulcerations around the ankle. Pulses are present but may be difficult to find because of edema. The foot may become cyanotic when dependent.

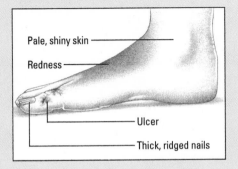

Pale, shiny skin

Redness

Ulcer

Thick, ridged nails

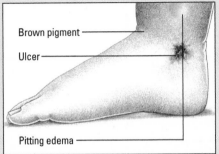

Brown pigment

Ulcer

Pitting edema

Strong or bounding pulsations usually occur in patients with conditions that cause increased cardiac output, such as hypertension, hypoxia, anemia, exercise, or anxiety. (See *Pulse waveforms*, page 32.)

A thrilling find

A heave, a lifting of the chest wall felt during palpation along the left sternal border, may mean right ventricular hypertrophy; over the left ventricular area, a ventricular aneurysm. A thrill, which is a palpable vibration, usually suggests valvular dysfunction.

Abnormal auscultation findings

A murmurlike sound of vascular (rather than cardiac) origin is called a *bruit*. If you hear a bruit during arterial auscultation, the patient may have occlusive arterial disease or an arteriovenous fistula. Various high cardiac output

(Text continues on page 34.)

Pulse waveforms

Pulse waveforms can be used to identify the type of an abnormal arterial pulse.

Weak pulse
A weak pulse is characterized by a decreased amplitude with a slower upstroke and down-stroke. Possible causes include increased peripheral vascular resistance, which can occur in cold weather or with severe heart failure, and decreased stroke volume, which can occur with hypovolemia or aortic stenosis.

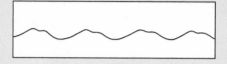

Bounding pulse
A bounding pulse has a sharp upstroke and downstroke with a pointed peak. The amplitude is elevated. Possible causes of a bounding pulse include increased stroke volume, which can occur with aortic insufficiency, or stiffness of arterial walls, which can occur with aging.

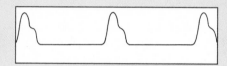

Pulsus alternans
Pulsus alternans is characterized by a regular, alternating pattern of a weak and a strong pulse. This pulse is associated with left-sided heart failure.

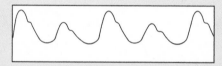

Pulsus bigeminus
Pulsus bigeminus is similar to pulsus alternans but occurs at irregular intervals. This pulse is caused by premature atrial or ventricular beats.

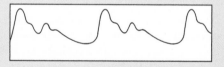

Pulsus paradoxus
Pulsus paradoxus is characterized by increases and decreases in amplitude associated with the respiratory cycle. Marked decreases occur when the patient inhales. Pulsus paradoxus is associated with pericardial tamponade, advanced heart failure, and constrictive pericarditis.

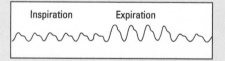

Inspiration   Expiration

Pulsus biferiens
Pulsus biferiens appears as an initial upstroke, a subsequent downstroke, and then another upstroke during systole. Pulsus biferiens is caused by aortic stenosis and aortic insufficiency.

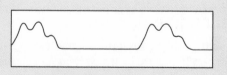

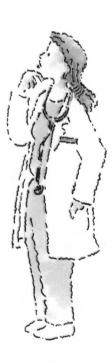

Interpreting cardiovascular assessment findings

A cluster of assessment findings may strongly suggest a particular cardiovascular disorder. In the chart below, column one shows groups of key signs and symptoms—those that compel the patient to seek medical attention. Column two shows related findings that you may discover during the health history and physical assessment. The patient may exhibit one or more of these findings. Column three shows the possible cause indicated by a cluster of these findings.

Key signs and symptoms	Related findings	Possible cause
• Dull or burning chest pain or a feeling of pressure, tightness, or heaviness that builds and fades gradually and may radiate to the abdomen, jaw, teeth, face, or left arm • Dyspnea, possibly with a sense of constriction around the larynx or upper trachea • Palpitations or skipped beats	• Family or personal history of coronary artery disease (CAD), atherosclerotic heart disease, stroke, diabetes, gout, or hypertension • History of obesity caused by excessive carbohydrate and saturated fat intake; smoking; lack of exercise; stress • Male over age 40; postmenopausal female • Precipitating factors, such as exertion, stress, hot or cold weather, and emotional turmoil • Anxiety, diaphoresis, tachycardia, transient crackles, paradoxical second heart sound (S_2) splitting • Blood pressure changes, possibly hypertension, particularly during an episode of chest pain	Angina pectoris
• Constricting, crushing, heavy-weightlike chest pain that occurs suddenly, may build to maximum intensity in a few minutes, and usually affects the central and substernal areas but isn't relieved by nitroglycerin • Dyspnea, possibly accompanied by orthopnea and cough • Fatigue and weakness • Palpitations or skipped beats	• Family or personal history of CAD, stroke, diabetes mellitus, gout, or hypertension • History of obesity, smoking, lack of exercise, stress, or angina • Anxiety, sense of impending doom • Nausea and vomiting • Diaphoresis, pallor or cyanosis • Tachycardia or bradycardia and weak pulse; arrhythmias • Normal or decreased blood pressure • Third (S_3) or fourth (S_4) heart sound, pericardial friction rub, or crackles	Acute myocardial infarction
• Exertional dyspnea • Cough • Dyspnea at rest (in advanced disease) • Orthopnea • Paroxysmal nocturnal dyspnea • Fatigue on exertion, accompanied by weakness • Tachycardia and skipped beats	• Use of pillows to improve breathing during sleep • Wheezing on inspiration and expiration • Nocturia • Anorexia, progressive weight gain, generalized edema, fatigue • Profuse diaphoresis, pallor or cyanosis • Frothy white or pink sputum • Heaving apical impulse • S_3 and S_4, basilar crackles	Left-sided heart failure

(continued)

Interpreting cardiovascular assessment findings *(continued)*

Key signs and symptoms	Related findings	Possible cause
• Dyspnea • Fatigue, in severe cases accompanied by weakness and confusion • Irregular heartbeat • Dependent edema that begins in the ankles and progresses to the legs and genitalia (initially subsides at night; later, doesn't) • Weight gain	• Anorexia, right upper abdominal discomfort, nausea, vomiting • History of left-sided heart failure, mitral or pulmonic valve stenosis, tricuspid insufficiency, pulmonary hypertension, or chronic obstructive pulmonary disease • Enlarged, tender, pulsating liver • Tricuspid insufficiency murmur • Ascites, splenomegaly • Jugular vein distention, tachycardia, S_3	Acute right-sided heart failure
• Paroxysmal nocturnal dyspnea accompanied by orthopnea • Fatigue • Palpitations • Possible edema and ascites	• Signs of heart failure, such as peripheral edema, basilar crackles, dyspnea, and tachycardia • Cardiac impulse displaced to the left • Systolic murmur, S_3 • Orthostatic hypotension	Cardiomyopathies
• Chest pain • Dyspnea • Fatigue or malaise • Weight loss	• Recent history of acute infection, surgery, instrumentation, dental work, drug abuse, abortion, or transurethral prostatectomy • History of rheumatic, congenital, or valvular heart disease • Intermittent fever, night sweats, chills • Petechiae on conjunctivae and buccal mucosa, splinter hemorrhages beneath nails, pallor or yellow-brown skin • Splenomegaly • Change in existing heart murmur or development of new murmur • Embolization to spleen, kidneys, brain, lungs, or peripheral vasculature • Osler's nodes, Roth's spots, and Janeway lesions	Subacute or acute bacterial endocarditis
• Dyspnea, paroxysmal nocturnal dyspnea • Fatigue, usually severe • Peripheral edema	• Female patient • History of mitral valve disease • Diastolic murmur at lower left sternal border that increases with inspiration, diastolic rumbling • Right ventricular lift • Ascites, hepatomegaly, jugular vein distention • Cyanosis during crying, poor feeding, and poor activity tolerance in a child	Tricuspid stenosis

conditions—such as anemia, hyperthyroidism, and pheochromocytoma—may also cause bruits. (See *Interpreting cardiovascular assessment findings*, pages 33 to 35.)

Interpreting cardiovascular assessment findings (continued)

Key signs and symptoms	Related findings	Possible cause
• Dyspnea on exertion or at rest • Orthopnea • Paroxysmal nocturnal dyspnea • Hemoptysis • Fatigue that worsens as exercise tolerance declines	• Female patient under age 45 • Recent bronchitis or upper respiratory tract infection that may worsen symptoms • History of rheumatic fever, congenital valve disorder, or tumor (myxoma) • Flushed cheeks • Lower left parasternal lift or heave • Tapping sensation over normal area of apical impulse • Middiastolic or presystolic thrill (or both) at apex • Small, weak pulse • Opening snap	Mitral stenosis
• Dyspnea on exertion • Fatigue • Possible peripheral edema	• History of congenital stenosis or rheumatic heart disease associated with other congenital heart defects, such as tetralogy of Fallot • Jugular vein distention • Hepatomegaly • Systolic murmur at left sternal border • Split S_2 with delayed or absent pulmonary component • Cyanosis during crying, poor feeding, and poor activity tolerance in a child	Pulmonic stenosis
• Dyspnea on exertion • Fatigue • Syncope • Chest pain	• Aging, history of congenital stenosis, rheumatic fever • Systolic murmur of right sternal border • Heart failure • Pulmonary edema	Aortic stenosis

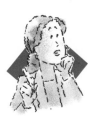

Quick quiz

1. Your patient's fingernails feel spongy upon palpation. This finding indicates:
    A.   chronic hypoxia.
    B.   bacterial infection.
    C.   an impending heart attack.
    D.   heart failure.

Answer: A. Spongy fingernails indicate clubbing, a sign that the patient suffers from chronic hypoxia due to a lengthy cardiovascular or respiratory disorder.

2.   When assessing an apical impulse in an obese patient, you should:

  A.   place the patient in a supine position.
  B.   have the patient lie on his right side.
  C.   have the patient lie on his left side.
  D.   have the patient sit up.

Answer: D. When an obese patient sits up, the heart sits closer to the anterior chest wall.

3.   Capillary refill time is normally:

  A.   1 to 3 seconds.
  B.   4 to 6 seconds.
  C.   7 to 10 seconds.
  D.   longer than 10 seconds.

Answer: A. Capillary refill time longer than 3 seconds is considered prolonged and indicates decreased perfusion.

4.   Upon examination, you find that your patient — a male, age 53 — has a forceful apical impulse. This finding:

  A.   suggests valvular disease.
  B.   indicates increased cardiac output.
  C.   suggests enlarged ventricles.
  D.   is normal in a middle-age patient.

Answer: B. A forceful apical impulse may indicate increased cardiac output.

5.   When performing arterial auscultation on a 35-year-old male patient, you hear a bruit over his femoral artery. Which of the following conditions wouldn't cause a bruit?

  A.   Anemia
  B.   Hypothyroidism
  C.   Hyperthyroidism
  D.   Pheochromocytoma

Answer: B. Hypothyroidism doesn't cause bruits. Bruits may result from occlusion of the artery or various other high cardiac output conditions, such as anemia, hyperthyroidism, and pheochromocytoma.

Scoring

☆☆☆ If you answered all five questions correctly, take a bow! You're a cardiovascular assessment star!

☆☆ If you answered four questions correctly, sensational! You're pumped with information!

☆ If you answered fewer than four questions correctly, keep at it! You're just getting the beat!

3

Cardiac auscultation

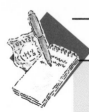

Just the facts

In this chapter, you'll learn:

♦ qualities to look for when choosing a stethoscope

♦ methods to improve your auscultation skills

♦ techniques to enhance heart sounds during auscultation.

A look at cardiac auscultation

The cardiovascular system requires more auscultation than any other body system. Gaining the skill necessary to detect cardiac abnormalities only comes after lots of practice. To understand auscultation findings, you'll need to use your knowledge of cardiac anatomy and physiology and also apply findings from other parts of the assessment.

Auscultation equipment

To perform auscultation, you'll need a stethoscope. The stethoscope picks up the sound of heart vibrations that are transmitted to the chest wall. Some vibrations are easy to hear; others are less distinct. The quality of your stethoscope influences how well you hear subtle differences in sounds. (See *Getting to know your stethoscope*, page 38.)

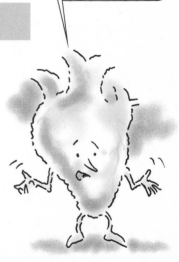

I know the cardiovascular system requires more auscultation than other body systems, but I can't help it if I'm high maintenance.

Getting to know your stethoscope

Before you begin to auscultate, familiarize yourself with all the parts of your stethoscope. Let's start at the bottom:
• The *chestpiece,* which rests on the patient's skin during auscultation, consists of either a *diaphragm,* a *bell,* or a combination of the two.
• The *stem* is a short metal tube that connects the chestpiece to the tubing. In some stethoscopes, the tubing hides the stem. The stem swivels to open either the diaphragm or the bell for auscultation.
• Flexible *tubing* connects the stem to the ear tubes. Some stethoscopes have only one tube (single lumen); others have two tubes (double lumen), which may be encased in a single shell.
• The metal *headset* contains the *binaurals* (ear tubes), ear tips, and *tension bar.* To loosen the headset, pull the ear tubes apart; to tighten it,

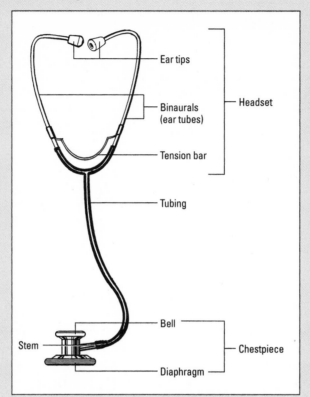

push them together, crossing them as you do so.
• Fitting snugly into the tubing, two inflexible *binaurals* transmit sound to your ears.

• The *ear tips,* which come in a variety of sizes and shapes, should fit snugly and comfortably inside your ears.

Choosing a stethoscope

To gain the most from your auscultation assessment, choose a stethoscope with both a diaphragm and a bell. The diaphragm transmits high-pitched sounds more clearly, while the bell transmits low-pitched sounds. You'll also use the bell for pediatric or thin patients, to listen around bandages, and to perform carotid assessment.

A flat, adult-sized diaphragm should be about 1⅜″ (3.5 cm) across. It should also be smooth, thin, and stiff

Buying a stethoscope

The first step in buying a stethoscope is to consider the situations in which you'll be using it. For example, do you work in a cardiac unit, a pediatrics facility, or an office setting? Each setting requires different features in a stethoscope. Stethoscopes labeled as cardiology stethoscopes transmit sound more accurately; however, you may not need such an advanced feature. After all, the more features a stethoscope has, the more expensive it will be. Also remember, no matter how sophisticated the stethoscope, the accuracy of the assessment depends on the skill of the person using it.

When making a choice, consider the following variations in chestpieces and tubing.

Chestpiece
• The chestpiece should have both a diaphragm and a bell.
• Some stethoscopes have a single-sided chestpiece, which functions like a bell when light pressure is applied and like a diaphragm with firmer pressure.
• If appropriate, choose an infant chestpiece (¾″ diameter) or a pediatric chestpiece (1″ diameter).

Tubing
• Single tubing provides adequate sound for basic assessments.
• Double tubing, which transmits sound through both tubes, is more sensitive and can yield more accurate auscultation findings. However, the sound of the two tubes rubbing together can be distracting, requiring both you and the patient to remain still.
• Double-lumen tubing provides the same sound as double tubing, with an added advantage: the outer shell keeps the two tubes from rubbing together, eliminating extraneous noise.
• Tubing length is mostly a matter of personal preference. Long tubing may dampen sound, although you probably won't notice the decrease. At the same time, long tubing may help you hear low-frequency sounds. When making a choice, consider how close you'll need to be to the patient during auscultation, how you'll carry the stethoscope (such as around your neck or in your pocket), and whether the strain of leaning over to listen with very short tubing would hurt your back.

enough to filter out low-frequency sounds. The bell should be about 1″ (2.5 cm) across and deep enough so that it doesn't fill with skin when you press it against the patient's chest wall. The tubing can range from 10″ to 15″ (25 to 38 cm) long, with a diameter of ⅛″ for shorter tubing and ³⁄₁₆″ for longer tubing. The earpieces should fit comfortably inside your ears and cover the external ear canals. Don't use a stethoscope that's too heavy; the excess weight can interfere with your ability to hear sounds accurately. (See *Buying a stethoscope*.)

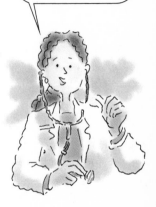

Not all stethoscopes are created equal. Make sure you choose the right stethoscope for your area of practice.

Becoming familiar with your stethoscope

To maximize the effectiveness of auscultation, practice holding the diaphragm and bell correctly. To listen with the diaphragm, either grasp the metal area between the bell and diaphragm with your thumb and index finger or place your fingertips on the rim of the bell. Then press firmly against the chest wall. Apply enough pressure so that a slight indentation remains on the skin after you remove the stethoscope.

Tender touch

When listening with the bell, use a lighter touch. Exerting too much pressure stretches the skin beneath the bell, causing it to act as a diaphragm and filter out low-pitched sounds. To use the bell, grasp the diaphragm's outer edges with your thumb and index finger and gently rest the bell on the chest wall. Look at the skin around the edges of the bell to make sure you aren't applying too much pressure. If you see signs of indentation, relax the downward pressure.

There's the rub

Also, remember to hold the chestpiece so that the tubing doesn't touch you or the patient. Rubbing against the tube can create sounds that interfere with auscultation.

Auscultation technique

Before you begin the auscultation, explain the procedure to the patient. Tell him to breathe normally, inhaling through the nose and exhaling through the mouth.

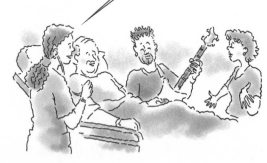

I know you're trying to cheer him up, but can you please keep it down a minute?

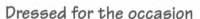

Preparing the patient

As you prepare to perform cardiac auscultation, make sure the room remains as quiet as possible. If the patient has any special equipment, such as oxygen or a suction device, perform auscultation with the equipment off, if possible.

Dressed for the occasion

Don't try to auscultate through clothing or surgical dressings; these items muffle heart sounds or make them inaudible. Instead, open the front of the patient's gown and drape him appropriately to limit the area exposed during auscultation. Make sure that the patient stays warm; muscle movement from shivering can interfere with hearing sounds clearly.

Set the stage

Have the patient lie on his back for the first part of the assessment. You may raise the head of the bed slightly if it makes the patient more comfortable. Stand on the patient's right side if you're right-handed, and on his left side if you're left-handed, so you can manipulate the stethoscope with your dominant hand.

Performing the assessment

To perform the assessment, first identify the sites where you'll auscultate: over the four heart valves and at Erb's point. (See *Auscultatory sequence*, page 42.)

Warming up the instrument

When you're ready to auscultate, warm the stethoscope between your hands. Remember to listen first with the diaphragm and then with the bell. Listen through several cardiac cycles to become accustomed to the sound, concentrating to hear any subtle changes.

Listen for the "dub"

To begin, use the diaphragm and auscultate at the aortic area where the second heart sound (S_2) is loudest. S_2 is best heard at the base of the heart at the end of ventricular systole. This sound corresponds to closure of the pulmonic and aortic valves and is generally described as sounding like "dub." It's a shorter, higher-pitched, louder sound than the first heart sound (S_1). When the pulmonic valve closes later than the aortic valve during inspiration, you'll hear a split S_2.

Listen for the "lub"

From the base of the heart, move to the pulmonic area, then to Erb's point, and then down to the tricuspid area. Next, move to the mitral area, where S_1 is loudest. S_1 is best heard at the apex of the heart. This sound corresponds to closure of the mitral and tricuspid valves and is generally described as sounding like "lub." Low-pitched and dull, S_1 occurs at the beginning of ventricular systole. It may be split if the mitral valve closes just before the tricuspid valve.

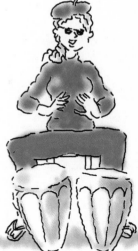

"Lub-dub, lub-dub." Now that's a tune a heart can dance to.

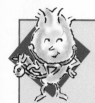

Location, location, location

Auscultatory sequence

When auscultating for heart sounds, place the stethoscope over the four different valve sites and at Erb's point. Follow the same auscultation sequence during every cardiovascular assessment:

• First place the stethoscope in the second intercostal space along the right sternal border, as shown. In the aortic area, blood moves from the left ventricle during systole, crossing the aortic valve and flowing through the aortic arch.

• Then move to the pulmonic area, located in the second intercostal space at the left sternal border. In the pulmonic area, blood ejected from the right ventricle during systole crosses the pulmonic valve and flows through the main pulmonary artery.

• Next, listen at Erb's point, located in the third intercostal space at the left sternal border. At Erb's point, you'll hear aortic and pulmonic sounds.

• At the fourth auscultation site, listen over the tricuspid area, which lies in the

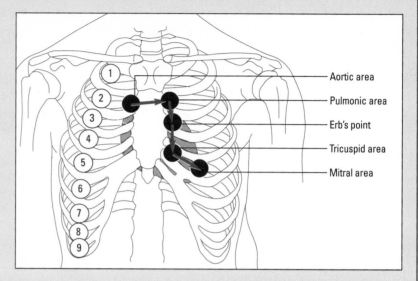

fifth intercostal space along the left sternal border. In the tricuspid area, sounds reflect blood movement from the right atrium across the tricuspid valve, filling the right ventricle during diastole.

• Finally, listen in the mitral area, located in the fifth intercostal space near the midclavicular line. (If the patient's heart is enlarged, the mitral area may be closer to the anterior axillary line.) In the mitral (apical) area, sounds represent blood flow across the mitral valve and left ventricular filling during diastole.

Feel the beat

Next, listen over the point of maximal impulse, which is usually found in the mitral area. To locate this point, have the patient shift slightly onto his left side into a left lateral decubitus position. This brings the apex of the heart closer to the chest wall. Look closely at the chest wall for pulsations. Then use your fingertips to feel for the pulsation (the apical pulse) between the fourth and sixth intercostal spaces, near the left midclavicular line. Listen here first with the diaphragm and then with the bell.

Expanding your horizons

When performing your assessment, keep in mind that heart valves transmit sound to specific *areas* of the precordium, not just to specific points. Because these areas overlap each other, focusing on the key sites discussed earlier can help you identify the sounds for each valve. However, in certain instances, such as if the patient has an enlarged heart, you'll need to broaden the area you auscultate. (See *Alternate auscultation areas*, page 44.)

After you've completed the auscultatory sequence with the patient lying down, have him sit up, if possible, while you complete the sequence a second time.

Enhancing auscultation findings

Auscultation of heart sounds can be difficult. Even with a stethoscope, the amount of tissue between the source of the sound and the outer chest wall can affect which sounds you hear. Fat, muscle, and air tend to reduce sound transmission. If a patient is obese, has a muscular chest wall, or has hyperinflated lungs, the sounds may seem distant and difficult to hear.

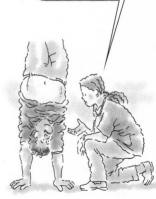

I appreciate your help, but this isn't the change in position I was talking about.

Change of scenery

If heart sounds seem distant, try placing the patient in an alternate position, which may enhance heart sound auscultation. (See *Alternate auscultation positions*, page 45.)

Going through the motions

If placing the patient in an alternate position doesn't amplify heart sounds, methods that change the flow of blood to the heart may help. For example, try auscultating while the patient stands, squats, holds his breath, or raises his legs while lying on his back. Another common technique is to have the patient cough several times or perform Valsalva's maneuver. Keep in mind that Valsalva's maneuver amplifies only systolic murmurs. In other instances, it can interfere with your auscultation efforts.

Breathing easy

Another method to enhance heart sounds is to have the patient take deep breaths. This slows the patient's respira-

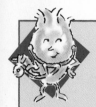

Location, location, location

Alternate auscultation areas

When a patient's heart is enlarged, heart sounds extend beyond the traditional auscultation sites. In these instances, broaden your auscultation assessment to include the areas shown in the illustration at right.

After you've completed your traditional auscultatory sequence, auscultate the alternative areas starting at the apex and working your way up:

• First, place the stethoscope in the left ventricular area, which is located from the second to the fifth intercostal space, and from the left sternal border to the left midclavicular line. This area increases in all directions if the patient has an enlarged left ventricle. Mitral and aortic murmurs and murmurs associated with hypertrophic obstructive cardiomyopathy are best heard here.

• Next, listen at the right ventricular area, located between the second and fifth intercostal spaces over the sternum. If the patient has a severely enlarged right ventricle, the area may extend to the point of maximal impulse. A right ventricular S_3 or S_4 and murmurs from tricuspid stenosis or insufficiency are heard here.

• Then move to the right atrial area, located along the right sternal border between the third and fifth intercostal spaces. If the patient's right atrium is severely enlarged, this area may extend beyond the right midclavicular line. This area is where the mur-

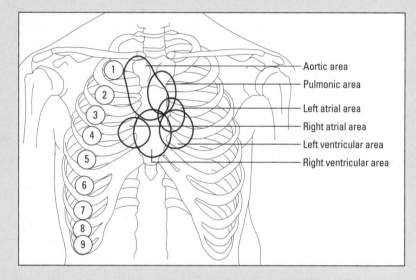

Aortic area
Pulmonic area
Left atrial area
Right atrial area
Left ventricular area
Right ventricular area

mur from tricuspid insufficiency is heard best.

• Next, listen at the left atrial area, located along the left sternal border, between the second and fourth intercostal spaces. Listen here for the murmur resulting from mitral insufficiency.

• Then move to the pulmonic area, located between the second and third intercostal spaces near the left side of the sternum. Listen here for murmurs from pulmonic stenosis and insufficiency and patent ductus arteriosus.

• Finally, listen in the aortic area, located from the right second intercostal space to the apex of the heart. This is where you'll hear murmurs from aortic stenosis and insufficiency.

tory rate, making it easier for you to differentiate between sounds heard during inspiration (reflecting events in the right side of the heart) and expiration (reflecting events occurring in the left side of the heart). Tell the patient that you'll raise your hand when you want him to inhale and that you'll lower your hand when you want him to exhale. Make sure, however, that the patient takes regular, even breaths. Breath holding could inadvertently trigger

Alternate auscultation positions

If heart sounds seem faint or undetectable, you may have to reposition the patient. Alternate positioning may enhance sounds or make them seem louder by bringing the heart closer to the chest's surface. Common alternate positions include a seated, forward-leaning position and the left lateral decubitus position. If these positions don't amplify heart sounds, try auscultating with the patient standing or squatting.

Forward-leaning position

Use the forward-leaning position when listening for high-pitched sounds related to semilunar valve problems, such as aortic and pulmonic valve murmurs. After helping the patient into this position, place the stethoscope's diaphragm over the aortic and pulmonic areas at the right and left second intercostal space.

Left lateral decubitus position

The left lateral decubitus position proves especially helpful when listening for low-pitched sounds related to atrioventricular valve problems, such as mitral valve murmurs and extra heart sounds. After helping the patient into this position, place the stethoscope's bell over the apical area.

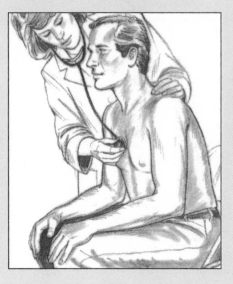 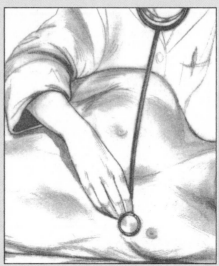

Valsalva's maneuver, which may alter auscultation findings.

Increasing the learning curve

Some patients—such as critically ill patients, elderly patients, children, and patients who don't speak English—present special challenges to the assessment process. (See *Considerations in special populations*, page 46.)

Considerations in special populations

When assessing a patient who is critically ill, is elderly or very young, or doesn't speak English, you may need to adjust your usual auscultation process. Apply these tips to help the assessment process proceed smoothly.

For a critically ill patient

• Ask for assistance to properly position the patient, especially if he has a ventilator, intra-aortic balloon pump (IABP), or Swan-Ganz catheter.
• Place a patient with left-sided heart failure in the left lateral position. This will bring the heart closer to the chest wall and make the point of maximal impulse easier to locate.
• To accentuate mitral and tricuspid murmurs, place the patient in a recumbent position.
• To amplify extraneous heart sounds (such as S_3 and S_4), place the patient in a left semilateral position.
• To amplify the sound of the tricuspid valve opening, have the patient sit up.
• If the patient has an IABP, briefly pause the balloon if the patient's condition allows. This will allow you to hear the patient's heart sounds without balloon assistance.

For an elderly patient

• Take into account that degenerative bony prominences can shift cardiac anatomy downward or laterally.

• Keep in mind that murmurs due to aging typically result from incompetent valves.
• Have the patient sit up and lean forward to accentuate murmurs from aortic or pulmonic regurgitation.
• Keep in mind that a patient with a memory disorder may become frightened or defensive if you lift his clothing for an assessment. Take time to orient him before you begin.

For a pediatric patient

• Be sure to use an appropriate-sized stethoscope. Most stethoscopes have an adapter for a smaller diaphragm.
• Know that murmurs in pediatric patients are typically associated with ventricular septal defects, patent ductus arteriosus, atrial septal defects, and mitral valve prolapse. Most of these murmurs are harmless and resolve over time.
• Take into account that exercise, crying, fever, and position change can accentuate murmurs.

For a non-English-speaking patient

• Approach the patient in a non-threatening manner.
• Use an interpreter, if possible.
• Demonstrate the assessment process on yourself before assessing the patient.
• Use drawings to enhance your explanation, if appropriate.
• Try to have the patient acknowledge his understanding before you begin.

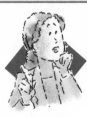

Quick quiz

1. To hear high-pitched heart sounds during an auscultation, use:

    A. the diaphragm.
    B. the bell.
    C. the diaphragm and the bell.
    D. a stethoscope with long, single tubing.

Answer: A. The diaphragm best amplifies high-pitched sounds, and the bell amplifies low-pitched sounds. For advanced auscultation, as well as better overall auscultation, stethoscopes with shorter tubing and a double lumen provide more clarity.

2. Begin your auscultation sequence by listening over:
   A. the tricuspid area.
   B. the pulmonic area.
   C. the aortic area.
   D. Erb's point.

Answer: C. Typically, you should begin the auscultation sequence over the aortic area. After listening through several cycles, inch across the chest to the pulmonic area, then down to Erb's point, then to the tricuspid area, and finally to the mitral area.

3. To locate the point of maximal impulse, have the patient:
   A. stand up.
   B. lie in a right lateral recumbent position.
   C. lie in a left lateral recumbent position.
   D. lie on his back with his head slightly elevated.

Answer: C. Have the patient turn slightly to the left, in a left lateral recumbent position. This brings the apex of the heart closer to the chest wall. After observing the chest wall for a rhythmic bulging, listen to the point of maximal impulse between the fourth and sixth intercostal spaces near the midclavicular line.

4. You may have difficulty hearing heart sounds in all of the following patients, except:
   A. an obese patient.
   B. a patient with hyperinflated lungs.
   C. a patient who's shivering.
   D. an anorexic patient.

Answer: D. Fat, air, and muscle may reduce sound transmission. Shivering or any other muscular movement during auscultation may interfere with sound transmission.

5. Which of the following techniques doesn't enhance heart sounds during auscultation?
   A. Having the patient squat or stand
   B. Having the patient drink water before auscultation
   C. Having the patient cough
   D. Having the patient breathe deeply

Answer: B. Having the patient drink water before auscultation doesn't enhance heart sounds. The other techniques can be used to either increase or decrease blood flow to the heart, which should enhance heart sounds.

6. Which technique is most helpful in auscultating for an aortic valve murmur?

    A. Having the patient lie in the left lateral position

    B. Having the patient sit up and lean forward

    C. Placing the patient in a recumbent position

    D. Listening with the bell of the stethoscope pressed firmly against the patient's chest

Answer: B. The forward-leaning position enhances high-pitched heart sounds that are related to semilunar valve problems, such as aortic valve murmurs.

Scoring

☆☆☆ If you answered all six questions correctly, bravo! You've aced auscultation.

  ☆☆ If you answered four or five questions correctly, great job! It sounds like you have an ear for assessment.

    ☆ If you answered fewer than four questions correctly, don't lose heart! Cardiac auscultation requires lots of practice.

Heart sound origins

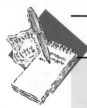

Just the facts

In this chapter, you'll learn:

♦ the origins of heart sounds

♦ characteristics used to describe heart sounds

♦ uses for electrocardiograms and phonocardiograms and their correlation with the heart's electrical activity

♦ proper documentation of heart sounds.

Understanding heart sound origins

Recall from previous chapters that the heart sounds you hear through the stethoscope during auscultation are generated by vibrations from the heart's walls and valves and from turbulent blood flow. Normally, the heart's walls and valves move in response to pressure and volume changes during the cardiac cycle.

Fab four

There are four distinct sounds:

☝ The first sound, S_1, occurs at the beginning of systole. It sounds like "lub."

✌ The second sound, S_2, is produced by the closing of the aortic and pulmonary valves. It sounds like "dub."

🖐 The third sound, S_3, is produced by the vibration that occurs when the ventricular walls are suddenly distended by the rush of blood from the heart's atria.

🖐 The fourth sound, S_4, is produced by atrial contraction and ventricular filling.

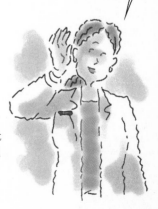

If you listen closely enough, you can hear four distinct heart sounds.

Basic heart sounds

Normally, the heart produces two basic heart sounds: S_1 and S_2. **(1)**

One for the money

S_1 is heard at the beginning of systole. It's generated by closure of the atrioventricular (AV) valves — the mitral and tricuspid valves. This sound is also associated with increased pressure within the ventricles that causes the moving valve leaflets and cord structures (the chordae tendineae) to slow down. (See *Visualizing the S_1 valves*.)

A normal heart produces two basic heart sounds — S_1 and S_2.

S_1 is heard at the beginning of systole and sounds like *lub*. S_2 is heard at the end of systole and sounds like *dub*.

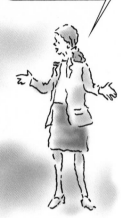

Visualizing the S_1 valves

The first heart sound (S_1) is associated with closure of the mitral and tricuspid valves (shown below) as well as with vibration of the ventricle walls caused by increasing pressure.

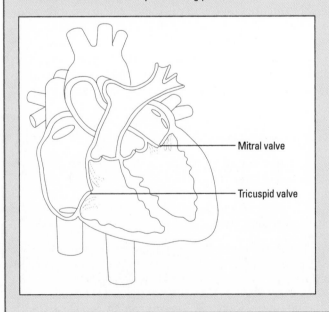

Mitral valve

Tricuspid valve

Visualizing the S₂ valves

The second heart sound (S_2) is associated with closure of the pulmonic and aortic valves (shown below).

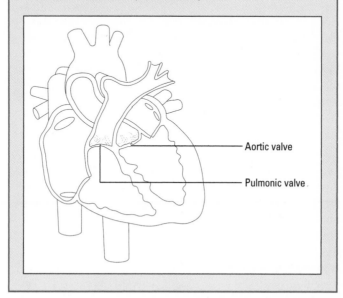

— Aortic valve

— Pulmonic valve

Two for the show

S_2 occurs at the end of ventricular systole, when ventricular pressure falls rapidly, causing a slight backflow of blood from the aorta and pulmonary artery. This decrease in ventricular pressure, temporary backflow of blood, and recoiling events cause the aortic and pulmonic valves to close. The vibrations associated with these events produce S_2, which marks the end of ventricular systole. **(2)** (See *Visualizing the S₂ valves*.)

Heart sound characteristics

Every heart sound has six different characteristics that need to be assessed during auscultation: location, intensity, duration, pitch, quality, and timing. If you keep these characteristics in mind each time you perform auscultation, your assessment of heart sounds will be complete and you'll be able to provide accurate and complete documentation. Also, because these terms are used universally,

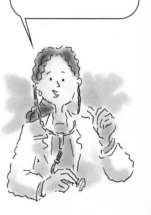

When auscultating for heart sounds, remember the six characteristics — location, intensity, duration, pitch, quality, and timing.

all health care professionals will be able to understand your auscultation findings.

Location

A sound's *location* is the anatomic area on the patient's chest wall where the sound is heard best. Bony structures and landmarks, such as the right and left midclavicular lines, are used to describe the exact location. For example, you might document that S_1 was heard best over the mitral area.

Intensity

Intensity refers to the loudness of the heart sound during auscultation. Usually, intensity is a somewhat subjective assessment that's based on experience. However, when abnormalities are present, intensity can be determined electronically using a phonocardiogram (PCG). A PCG measures and records the amplitude of the sound's vibrations and allows comparison of the sounds heard during auscultation to the heart's electrical activity recorded on the patient's electrocardiogram (ECG).

It's all relative

Keep in mind that heart sound intensity is related to the pressures generated and the blood flow velocity within the heart. It's also related to the patient's size, body build, and chest configuration. For example, a slender patient has a thinner chest wall, which allows sounds to be transmitted more easily than they would be through an obese patient's chest wall. (Recall that intensity = loudness, so if a sound is transmitted more easily, the loudness, or intensity, of the heart sound is heard without any interference.) What's more, certain interferences, such as pericardial fluid or the lung tissue of a patient with emphysema, can also diminish the amplitude of heart sounds.

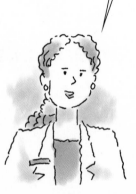

Keep in mind that heart sound intensity is related to such factors as the patient's size, body build, and chest configuration.

Duration

Duration refers to the length of time the heart sound is heard; it can be described as either short or long. Remember, heart sounds are brief vibrations that mark the beginning and end of systole. A sound's duration affects whether you hear it as a click, a snap, or a murmur. For example, murmurs are longer vibrations that are usually associated with blood flow during systole or diastole.

Pitch

The *pitch* of a heart sound is determined by the frequency of its vibrations. High-frequency sounds (like the notes of a piccolo) are best heard with the diaphragm of the stethoscope; low-frequency sounds (like the notes of a tuba) are best heard with the bell of the stethoscope.

Quality

The *quality* of a heart sound refers to the type of noise produced. It's determined by the combination of its frequencies. Such words as *sharp, dull, booming, machine-like, rumbling, snapping, blowing, harsh,* and *musical* can be used to describe the quality of heart sounds.

Timing

The *timing* of a heart sound refers to when it's heard during the cardiac cycle — that is, during systole or diastole.

Depolarization and repolarization

The heart can't pump unless an electrical stimulus occurs first. As electrical impulses are transmitted, cardiac cells go through cycles of depolarization and repolarization. This sequential and rhythmic process is referred to as the heart's *electrical activity*. Electrical activity occurs at the cellular level in every contractile cell of the myocardium. (See *Understanding the depolarization-repolarization cycle*, page 54.)

Depolarization

Initially, the contractile cardiac cells are polarized (in a resting state). *Depolarization* begins when the cell membranes become permeable and sodium ions flow into the cell.

Memory jogger

To remember which part of the stethoscope to use to hear which types of sounds, think: **Di-high; Bell-low.**

The **diaphragm** is used to hear **high**-pitched sounds, and the **bell** is used to hear **low** sounds.

Memory jogger

To remember the difference between depolarization and repolarization, keep in mind that **Re**polarization is an attempt to get back to the **Re**sting state (calcium ions move in; potassium ions move out).

Understanding the depolarization-repolarization cycle

The illustration below can help you understand the events that occur during the depolarization-repolarization cycle.

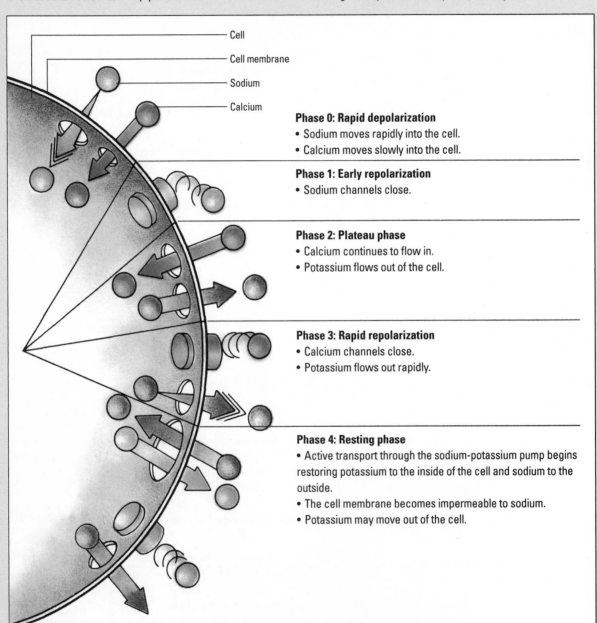

Cell

Cell membrane

Sodium

Calcium

Phase 0: Rapid depolarization
- Sodium moves rapidly into the cell.
- Calcium moves slowly into the cell.

Phase 1: Early repolarization
- Sodium channels close.

Phase 2: Plateau phase
- Calcium continues to flow in.
- Potassium flows out of the cell.

Phase 3: Rapid repolarization
- Calcium channels close.
- Potassium flows out rapidly.

Phase 4: Resting phase
- Active transport through the sodium-potassium pump begins restoring potassium to the inside of the cell and sodium to the outside.
- The cell membrane becomes impermeable to sodium.
- Potassium may move out of the cell.

Repolarization

When a cell is fully depolarized, it attempts to return to its resting state. This is known as *repolarization.*

Repolarization begins when calcium ions move into the cell and potassium ions begin to move out of the cell. Then, the sodium-potassium pump forces the accumulated intracellular sodium and calcium ions out of the cell while the lost potassium is restored to the cell, completing repolarization. The cell is polarized to its original ionic state, and the myocardium relaxes.

The ECG

Heart sounds are produced by mechanical events that occur in response to an electrical impulse originating in the sinoatrial (SA) node. This electrical impulse travels through the myocardium, activating the atria and ventricles. An ECG reflects all of the electrical activity (the depolarization-repolarization cycle) and documents the timing and amplitude of the heart's electrical activity from the atria to the ventricles.

It's electric...

Keep in mind that an ECG represents electrical activity only, not actual pumping of the heart. It's a valuable diagnostic tool that's now a routine part of every cardiovascular evaluation and should be included in the patient's chart. (See *What the ECG strip shows,* page 56.)

ECGs help identify primary conduction abnormalities, arrhythmias, cardiac hypertrophy, pericarditis, electrolyte imbalances, and the site and extent of myocardial infarction.

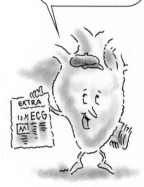

Read all about it! An ECG can tell you all about my timing and amplitude.

Components of the ECG

The first wave in an ECG occurs when the SA node fires and the impulse spreads through the atria. The P wave, part of the ECG waveform, represents atrial depolarization. Atrial contraction is stimulated by, and closely follows, atrial depolarization.

What the ECG strip shows

Here's a sample of the components of a normal electrocardiogram (ECG) waveform.

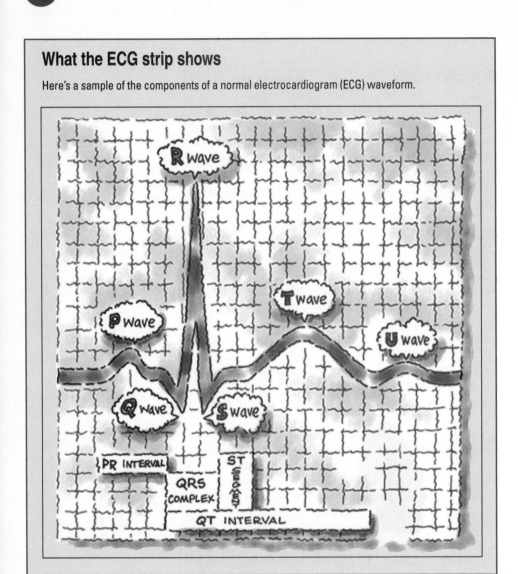

Next is the QRS

After the P wave, electrical depolarization of the ventricles occurs, producing the QRS complex. Atrial repolarization isn't seen in the ECG because it's hidden in the PR segment and the QRS complex.

On to the T wave

Next, during ventricular repolarization, the ventricles relax. This is represented by the T wave on the ECG.

In between it's the PR interval

The impulse travels through the AV node, the bundle of His, the bundle branches, and the Purkinje fibers before the ventricles contract. The time between atrial depolarization and ventricular depolarization is recorded on the ECG as the PR interval. It begins at the onset of the P wave and lasts until the onset of the QRS complex. The PR interval correlates with the time interval between atrial contraction and ventricular contraction.

Relationship to S_1 and S_2

S_1 and S_2 directly correlate with a patient's ECG. S_1 normally occurs just after the QRS complex, and S_2 occurs at the end of the T wave. (See *Finding S_1 and S_2 on the ECG*.)

Finding S_1 and S_2 on the ECG

The first heart sound (S_1) and the second heart sound (S_2) directly correlate with a patient's electrocardiogram (ECG). S_1 occurs just after the QRS complex, and S_2 occurs at the end of the T wave, as shown below.

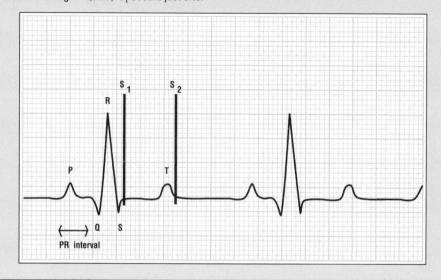

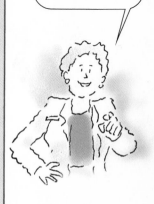

Just remember, S_1 occurs just after the QRS complex and S_2 occurs at the end of the T wave.

Documenting heart sounds

Each heart sound must be thoroughly documented. By including information about each of the six heart sound characteristics, you can precisely describe every heart sound, whether normal or abnormal. You can document what you heard, where you heard it, how you heard it, and when you heard it. Information about your patient's history can also be a valuable part of heart sound documentation. Consider documenting:
• family history of murmurs or other abnormal heart sounds
• other symptoms present, such as cyanosis, distended neck veins, and abnormal breath sounds.

Document what you heard, where you heard it, how you heard it, and when you heard it, so that others can recognize changes in the patient's heart sounds.

Let's be practical

Although a PCG is one method of graphically representing and documenting heart sounds, it isn't routinely used for every patient; moreover, it requires expensive equipment. Therefore, describing the location, intensity, duration, pitch, quality, and timing is a more practical method of documenting heart sounds.

The good of it all

Complete documentation provides other health care professionals with invaluable information that may help them recognize subtle changes in the patient's heart sounds.

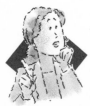

Quick quiz

1.   After auscultating for a patient's heart sounds, you document that S_1 was high rather than low. Which characteristic does this describe?
    A.   Location
    B.   Duration
    C.   Pitch
    D.   Quality

Answer: C. Pitch refers to the frequency of vibrations. Usually, the frequency of sounds may be described as high or low.

2. When you're describing the loudness of a patient's heart sound, you're referring to which characteristic?

    A. Pitch
    B. Intensity
    C. Quality
    D. Duration

Answer: B. Intensity refers to the sound's loudness.

3. Which time interval on the ECG correlates with the time interval between atrial depolarization and ventricular depolarization?

    A. PR interval
    B. QRS complex
    C. QT interval
    D. ST segment

Answer: A. The PR interval is the time between atrial depolarization and ventricular depolarization.

4. S_1 directly correlates with a patient's ECG. S_1 normally occurs:

    A. just after the P wave.
    B. after the QRS complex.
    C. at the end of the T wave.
    D. during the Q wave.

Answer: B. S_1 normally occurs just after the QRS complex.

5. S_2 directly correlates with a patient's ECG. S_2 normally occurs:

    A. just after the P wave.
    B. after the QRS complex.
    C. at the end of the T wave.
    D. during the Q wave.

Answer: C. S_2 normally occurs at the end of the T wave.

6. The characteristic that describes when you hear the heart sound during the cardiac cycle, such as during systole or diastole, is referred to as:

    A.   duration.
    B.   quality.
    C.   location.
    D.   timing.

Answer: D. Timing of a heart sound refers to when it's heard during the cardiac cycle.

Scoring

✰✰✰ If you answered all six questions correctly, dynamite! You obviously know the dynamics of heart sounds and can listen for them with ease.

✰✰ If you answered four or five questions correctly, keep going! You've got heart and you know what it takes to understand this chapter.

✰ If you answered fewer than four questions correctly, don't stress! It sounds like you might just need a refresher.

S₁ and S₂ heart sounds

Just the facts

In this chapter, you'll learn:

♦ components of S_1 and S_2

♦ differences between S_1 and S_2

♦ the best way to describe S_1 and S_2

♦ implications of abnormal S_1 and S_2 splits.

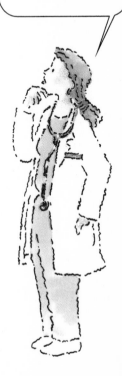

Understanding normal heart sounds gives you the basis for listening to other heart sounds.

A closer look at S₁ and S₂

A normal functioning heart produces two basic heart sounds: S_1 and S_2. S_1 results from the closing of the mitral and tricuspid valves. It indicates the beginning of systole and is the *lub* of the *lub-dub* sequence. S_2 results from the closing of the pulmonic and aortic valves. It indicates the end of systole and the beginning of diastole and creates a *dub* sound. Becoming familiar with normal heart sounds will help you note variations or abnormal heart sounds.

First heart sound, S₁

S_1 is produced by three actions:

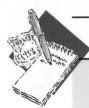 movement of blood within the ventricles

cardiac vibrations from the ventricle walls

closing of the mitral and tricuspid valves. **(3)**

Two in one

Occasionally, two components of S_1 are audible. Expiration makes them easier to hear. **(4)** The first component,

Location, location, location

Auscultating for S₁, M₁, and T₁

To listen to the first heart sound (S₁) and the mitral component (M₁), place your stethoscope over the mitral area, which is located in the fifth intercostal space at the midclavicular line. To hear the tricuspid component (T₁), if it's audible, place your stethoscope over the tricuspid area, located between the fourth and fifth intercostal spaces at the left lower sternal border.

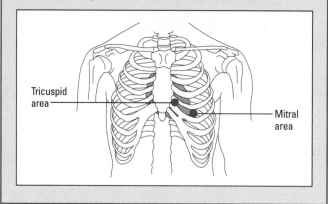

Tricuspid area

Mitral area

Valves involved in S₁

The valves involved in the first heart sound (S₁) are the tricuspid and mitral valves. S₁ is also caused by the movement of blood within the ventricles and the subsequent vibration of the ventricle walls.

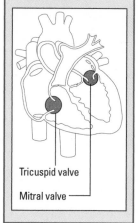

Tricuspid valve

Mitral valve

referred to as M₁, is associated with closure of the mitral valve; the second component, T₁, is associated with closure of the tricuspid valve. (See *Valves involved in S₁*.)

One step ahead

The mitral and tricuspid valves both close at the beginning of ventricular systole. The mitral valve usually closes slightly before the tricuspid valve. However, M₁ and T₁ are usually perceived as a single sound, called S₁. Most times, only the first heart sound (S₁) is heard because M₁ and T₁ are separated by a 20-millisecond, or shorter, pause that the human ear hears as one sound. (See *Auscultating for S₁, M₁, and T₁*.)

Characteristics of S₁

S₁ is usually heard best near the heart's apex over the mitral area at the lower left sternal border. Characteristics of this sound include:

- intensity directly related to the force of ventricular contraction and the PR interval on the electrocardiogram (ECG)
- shorter PR intervals, causing the mitral and tricuspid leaflets to open more widely at the onset of ventricular contraction
- slower heart rate that produces more intense vibrations when the leaflets close, causing a louder S$_1$
- longer duration than S$_2$
- high pitch that's heard best with the diaphragm of the stethoscope
- timing that coincides with the beginning of ventricular systole and a palpable carotid pulse **(5)**
- S$_1$ occurring just after the QRS complex in the ECG waveform. (See *S$_1$ and normal S$_1$ split on PCG and ECG*, page 64.)

Normal S$_1$ split

As you move the stethoscope from the mitral area toward the tricuspid area, without losing track of S$_1$, the M$_1$ and T$_1$ components of S$_1$ may become evident. T$_1$ trails M$_1$ slightly and is softer; it's heard best near the left sternal border. The timing of M$_1$ and T$_1$ with the QRS complex remains the same. The characteristics of the normally split S$_1$ into M$_1$ and T$_1$ are the same. **(6)** (See *Tips for hearing S$_1$ sounds*.)

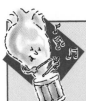

Now hear this!

Tips for hearing S$_1$ sounds

Auscultate for heart sounds with the patient in the left lateral decubitus, supine, and seated positions. For the first heart sound (S$_1$), the diaphragm and bell of the stethoscope should be used in an alternating fashion.

S$_1$ solutions
If S$_1$ is difficult to identify, palpate for the carotid pulse while performing auscultation.

S$_1$ will occur just before you feel the carotid pulse. Also, S$_1$ can be enhanced by sympathetic stimulation, such as that provided by a brief period of exercise.

For the mitral component (M$_1$) and the tricuspid component (T$_1$), auscultating the patient during expiration may make the sounds more audible.

S₁ and normal S₁ split on PCG and ECG

The first heart sound (S₁) occurs immediately after the QRS complex, as shown below.

Phonocardiogram (PCG) and electrocardiogram (ECG) showing S₁

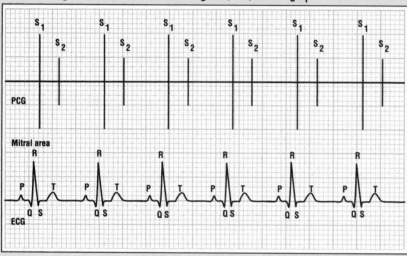

Let's split

In a normal S₁ split, the mitral (M₁) and tricuspid (T₁) components have the same timing as S₁. M₁ occurs slightly before T₁. The second heart sound (S₂) occurs immediately after the T wave.

PCG and ECG showing normal S₁ split

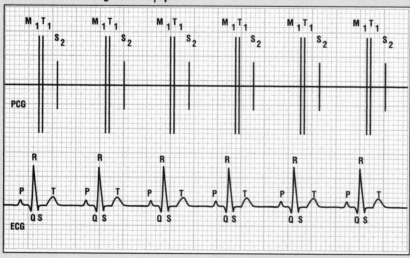

Abnormal S₁ split

The normal M_1-T_1 split heard over the tricuspid area widens when electrical activation and contraction of the right ventricle are delayed. Such a delay causes delayed tricuspid valve closure, thus causing a widening interval between M_1 and T_1. **(7)**

Opened wide

The widened interval between M_1 and T_1 is an abnormal S_1 split that may be referred to as a *widened S_1 split*. Widened S_1 splits are associated with complete right bundle-branch block (RBBB), left ventricular ectopic beats, tricuspid stenosis, atrial septal defect, and Ebstein's anomaly. (See *Auscultating for abnormal S_1 split*.)

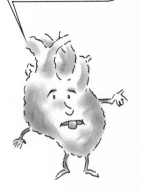

If you hear a widened S₁ split, then I may have right bundle-branch block, left ventricular ectopic beats, tricuspid stenosis, atrial septal defect, or Ebstein's anomaly.

Location, location, location

Auscultating for abnormal S₁ split

To auscultate for an abnormal first heart sound (S_1) split, place the stethoscope over the tricuspid area. You may hear a slight delay in the tricuspid component (T_1).

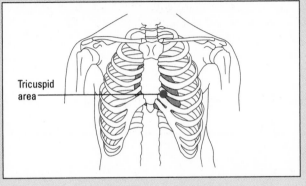

Tricuspid area

Second heart sound, S_2

S_2 is produced by the cardiac vibrations caused by the closing of the aortic and pulmonic valves as well as the sudden deceleration of blood in the aorta and pulmonary artery.

Two components: A_2 and P_2

S_2 is usually louder than S_1 at the heart's base and usually slightly higher in pitch than S_1 at the heart's apex. S_2, like S_1, has two basic components: the aortic component (A_2) and the pulmonic component (P_2). Both of these valves close at the end of ventricular systole. Normally, the aortic valve closes slightly ahead of the pulmonic valve because closing pressure is higher in the aorta than in the pulmonary artery. Therefore, A_2 usually occurs earlier and is louder than P_2. **(8)** (See *Valves involved in S_2.*)

Splitting sounds

When the right and left ventricles contract at slightly different times, the sounds are most commonly noted as a *split S_2*. This split isn't abnormal but, occasionally, it can indicate an abnormality such as enlargement of one of the ventricles.

Characteristics of S_2

S_2 is usually heard best near the heart's base, over the pulmonic area or over Erb's point. (See *Auscultating for S_2, A_2, and P_2.*)

Other characteristics of S_2 include:
* intensity directly relating to the amount of closing pressure in the aorta and pulmonary artery
* slightly shorter duration than S_1
* high pitch that's heard best with the diaphragm of the stethoscope
* booming quality
* timing coinciding with the end of ventricular systole. **(9)**

Normal S_2 split

The normal splitting of S_2 into the A_2 and P_2 components is heard best during inspiration over the pulmonic area. A

Valves involved in S_2

When you hear the second heart sound (S_2), you're listening to the closing of the aortic and pulmonic valves, shown below.

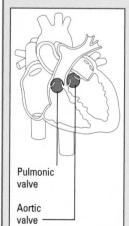

Pulmonic valve

Aortic valve

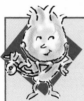

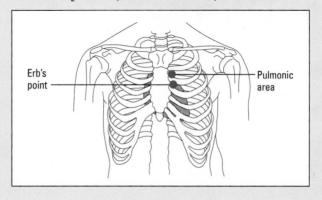

Location, location, location

Auscultating for S₂, A₂, and P₂

To hear both components of the second heart sound (S₂), listen carefully with the diaphragm of the stethoscope over the pulmonic area and Erb's point. The aortic component (A₂) is usually louder than the pulmonic component (P₂) over the pulmonic area, located at the left second intercostal space; however, if intense enough, it can be heard over the entire precordium. P₂, which is softer than A₂, is usually heard best over the pulmonic area.

Erb's point

Pulmonic area

normal S₂ split sounds like "lub/dubdub." Remember, inspiration reduces the intrathoracic pressure in the pulmonary artery. This decrease in pressure causes an increase in venous return to the right side of the heart. This increased venous return delays emptying of the right ventricle, prolonging right ventricular ejection time, and delays closure of the pulmonic valve.

Simultaneous split

A simultaneous decrease in blood flow to the heart's left side results in a shorter left ventricular ejection time, contributing to the S₂ split. Thus, a normal S₂ split is heard during inspiration. The two sounds normally fuse during expiration. (See *Respiratory changes in normal S₂ split on PCG and ECG*, page 68.) **(10)**

Respiratory changes in normal S_2 split on PCG and ECG

Normal second heart sound (S_2) splits are heard best during inspiration. As the patient begins to exhale, the S_2 split becomes narrower until it fuses together at expiration. These changes can be seen on the phonocardiogram (PCG) and electrocardiogram (ECG) representation below.

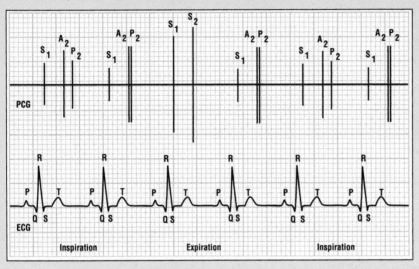

Changes in A_2 and P_2 intensity

While listening to S_2, you must determine the intensity of the A_2 and P_2 components. Also, note the duration of the A_2-P_2 interval and its relationship to the respiratory cycle. **(11)**

Under pressure

You should also document the S_2 split, noting whether the A_2-P_2 interval increases or decreases during inspiration and expiration. The intensity of A_2 and P_2 changes proportionally with the difference in pressure gradients across the closed aortic and pulmonic valves. For example, P_2 may be louder than normal in conditions associated with elevated pulmonary artery diastolic pressure, as occurs in some patients with heart failure, mitral stenosis, pulmonary hypertension, Eisenmenger's syndrome, or other congenital heart diseases. When P_2 increases in intensity, it's sometimes heard over the mitral area and along the left sternal border. **(12)**

Tense situation

A_2 intensity increases when diastolic pressure in the aorta increases. **(13)** This commonly happens during exercise; during states of excitement such as extreme fear; in hyperkinetic conditions, such as thyrotoxicosis, fever, and pregnancy; and in systemic hypertension. However, if the patient has left ventricular decompensation, ventricular relaxation is slower, and the pressure gradients may not be great enough to produce an accentuated A_2.

> My A_2 intensity increases not only during exercise but also during states of excitement, in hyperkinetic conditions, and in systemic hypertension.

In contrast

Conversely, A_2 intensity may be diminished in conditions that alter the development of diastolic pressure gradients, such as aortic insufficiency and hypotension. **(14)** A_2 intensity also decreases when ventricular dysfunction is present, such as after an acute myocardial infarction. In this condition, P_2 may become louder if pulmonary artery pressure rises and systemic pressure falls. A_2 is also softer or absent when aortic valve motion is restricted, as in severe aortic stenosis.

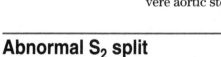

Abnormal S_2 split

Abnormal splitting is related to valvular dysfunction, alterations in blood flow to or from the ventricles, or both. These changes may cause the normal S_2 split to be absent during both phases of the respiratory cycle. Thus, only a single S_2 is heard over Erb's point. In another case, the split sounds may persist through inspiration and expiration with little or no respiratory variation. **(15)**

Noticeable changes

The split sounds may also be heard inconsistently on expiration. The A_2-P_2 intervals vary, as do the intensities of A_2 and P_2 during the respiratory cycle. **(16)** Changes in S_2 splits are usually most noticeable at the beginning of inspiration and expiration.

Absent S_2 split

The P_2 component may not be heard during auscultation over Erb's point in the patient with severe pulmonic stenosis. Consequently, S_2 remains a single sound during inspiration and expiration. A normal S_2 split may also be absent if the A_2 sound masks the P_2 sound or vice versa—for example, when one sound is significantly louder than the other, making splitting inaudible. This phenomenon occurs in patients with pulmonary hypertension. In contrast, systemic hypertension causes A_2 to be delayed and to fuse with P_2 during inspiration. In a patient with an increased anteroposterior chest dimension, the P_2 intensity may be so diminished that only A_2 is audible.

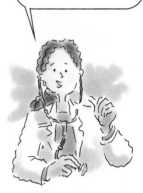

A normal S_2 split may be absent in patients with severe pulmonic stenosis, pulmonary hypertension, or increased anteroposterior chest dimension.

Persistent S_2 split

A persistent S_2 split occurs when A_2 and P_2 don't fuse into one sound during expiration. Rather, the split sounds persist throughout inspiration and expiration, even though some respiratory variation in the intensity of A_2 and P_2 is heard. **(17)** This persistent A_2-P_2 splitting during expiration usually results from mitral insufficiency or ventricular septal defect (VSD), which is heard as an early A_2. Atrial septal defect or dilation of the pulmonary artery may be heard as a late P_2. (See *Persistent S_2 split on PCG and ECG.*)

Narrow-minded

Early aortic valve closure is associated with shortened left ventricular systole, which occurs in patients with mitral insufficiency, VSDs, or cardiac tamponade. Delayed pulmonic valve closure occurs when right ventricular systole is prolonged from structural or physiologic changes or abnormalities, such as in patients with chronic pulmonary hypertension. In these patients, the A_2-P_2 split is heard. The split persists through inspiration and expiration, but the interval between the A_2 and P_2 components is narrowed as compared to the persistent S_2 split. **(18)**

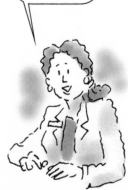

A persistent S_2 split may be due to mitral insufficiency or a VSD.

Delayed relay

Another cause of persistent A_2-P_2 splitting throughout expiration is delayed electrical activation of the right ventricle, which delays P_2. This phenomenon is commonly found in patients with RBBB, left ventricular epicardial pacing, or left ventricular ectopic beats.

Persistent S₂ split on PCG and ECG

In a persistent second heart sound (S₂) split, the aortic (A₂) and pulmonic (P₂) components don't fuse during inspiration or expiration. Although the components persist, their intensity may decrease with inspiration and increase with expiration, as shown on the phonocardiogram (PCG) and electrocardiogram (ECG) representation below.

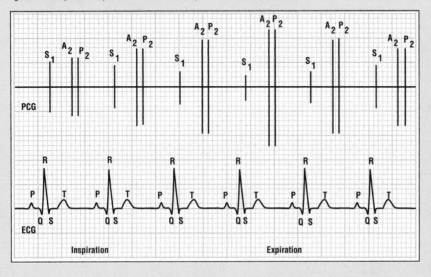

Widened S₂ split

Widened S₂ split may occur during inspiration or expiration. When it occurs during inspiration, it may indicate delayed activation of a contraction or emptying of the right ventricle, resulting in a delayed closing of the pulmonic valve. Widened S₂ split that varies with inspiration is commonly seen in patients with constrictive pericarditis, pulmonic stenosis, or RBBB.

On the outs

Widened S₂ splits during expiration occur as a result of delayed right or left ventricular ejection times. A delayed electrical activation of the right ventricle, resulting in a prolonged right ventricular ejection time, produces expiratory A₂-P₂ splits that are widened and persist even when the patient is seated. **(19)** Widened expiratory A₂-P₂ split from prolonged right ventricular ejection time occurs in patients with atrial septal defects, acute or severe pulmonary hypertension secondary to massive pulmonary emboli, or pulmonic stenosis. The P_2 component may not be audible at all in patients with severe pulmonic stenosis. A widened expiratory P_2 split from a delayed left ventricular ejection time may occur in patients with severe mitral insufficiency.

Fix-ation

A widened, fixed S_2 split doesn't change with respiration and is associated with the lungs' ability to receive blood volume and the decreased resistance that accompanies that volume. **(20)** Wide, fixed splitting occurs when the output of the right ventricle is greater than that of the left ventricle, thus causing a delay in the closing of the pulmonic valve. This phenomenon occurs in patients with idiopathic dilation of the pulmonary artery or large atrial septal defects. A widened, fixed S_2 split may also occur in patients with severe right-sided heart failure when there's little or no increase in right ventricular stroke volume after inspiration or in patients with a VSD with left-to-right shunting. (See *Widened, fixed S₂ split on PCG and ECG.*)

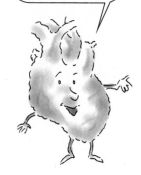

During expiration, widened S_2 splits may occur as a result of delayed right or left ventricular ejection times.

Widened, fixed S₂ split on PCG and ECG

Similar to persistent second heart sound (S_2) splits, widened, fixed S_2 splits don't fuse during inspiration or expiration. However, the S_2 split is widened, as shown on the phonocardiogram (PCG) and electrocardiogram (ECG) representation below.

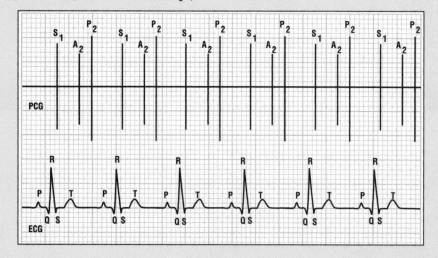

Paradoxical S_2 split

In a paradoxical, or reversed, S_2 split, P_2 precedes A_2, and the split sounds are heard during expiration instead of inspiration. **(21)** This phenomenon is almost always caused by delayed aortic valve closure. If A_2 is delayed during expiration, it may follow P_2, causing an S_2 split; if A_2 is delayed during inspiration, A_2 and P_2 fuse because inspiration normally delays P_2, causing S_2 to be heard as a single sound during inspiration instead of a normally split sound. **(22)** (See *Paradoxical S_2 split on PCG and ECG*.)

What's the delay?

Delayed A_2 is most commonly seen in patients with delayed electrical activation of the left ventricle caused by left bundle-branch block (LBBB). LBBB may delay closure of the aortic valve, which normally closes first. This delay causes the pulmonic valve to close first, so that the

Paradoxical S_2 split on PCG and ECG

Unlike normal second heart sound (S_2) splits, paradoxical S_2 splits occur during expiration rather than during inspiration because the aortic component (A_2), rather than the pulmonic component (P_2), is delayed, as shown on the phonocardiogram (PCG) and electrocardiogram (ECG) representation below. During inspiration, the components fuse together into one sound, S_2.

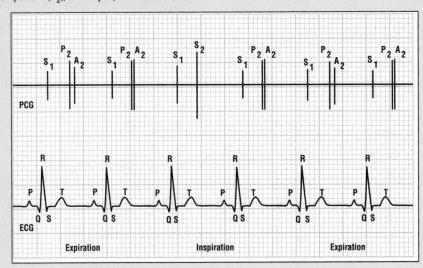

split is reversed and consists of P_2-A_2. LBBB is also associated with right ventricular endocardial pacing and premature right ventricular contractions, as in Wolff-Parkinson-White syndrome.

I can't hear you!

Paradoxical S_2 splits may also be caused by prolonged left ventricular systole, resulting from prolonged left ventricular ejection time. In this case, increased left ventricular stroke volume or increased resistance to left ventricular ejection may cause left ventricular pressure overload.

Left ventricular overload from increased left ventricular stroke volume is commonly seen in aortic insufficiency and patent ductus arteriosus. However, the paradoxical split is rarely heard. Left ventricular overload caused by increased pulmonary resistance, usually because of left-sided heart failure, commonly occurs in patients with systemic hypertension and hypertrophic cardiomyopathy. Aortic stenosis may also lead to paradoxical splitting of A_2 and P_2; however, if the stenosis is severe, the A_2 component may not be audible.

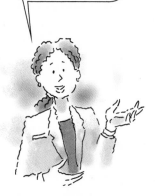

If aortic stenosis is severe, the A_2 of the paradoxical S_2 split may not be audible.

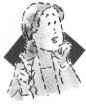

Quick quiz

1. When auscultating a patient's heart, you note a persistent S_2 split. This sound indicates that:

A. the normal S_2 split is absent.
B. closure of the pulmonic valve is early.
C. the aortic and pulmonic components don't fuse together.
D. closure of the aortic valve is delayed.

Answer: C. Persistent S_2 split occurs when the aortic and pulmonic components don't fuse into one sound during expiration. Rather, the split sounds persist throughout inspiration and expiration. Persistent S_2 split may also occur if the closure of the aortic valve is early or if the closure of the pulmonic valve is delayed.

2. Delayed closing of the tricuspid valve causes:
  A.   normal S_1 split.
  B.   widened S_1 split.
  C.   absent S_2 split.
  D.   widened, fixed S_2 split.

Answer: B. Normally, the tricuspid valve closes after the aortic valve. When closing of the tricuspid valve is delayed, a widened S_1 split results.

3. Which of the following conditions can be heard best during inspiration?
  A.   Paradoxical S_2 split
  B.   Persistent S_2 split
  C.   Normal S_2 split
  D.   Widened S_2 split

Answer: C. Normal S_2 splits are heard best during inspiration.

4. You're auscultating a healthy 35-year-old male for S_1 and S_2. When you hear the first heart sound, S_1, you're hearing the:
  A.   movement of blood within the atria.
  B.   cardiac vibrations from the atrial walls.
  C.   closing of the mitral and tricuspid valves.
  D.   closing of the aortic and pulmonic valves.

Answer: C. S_1 is produced by the closing of the mitral and tricuspid valves. S_1 is also produced by the movement of blood and vibrations within the ventricles.

5. In a patient with a paradoxical or reversed S_2 split, which valve is delayed?
  A.   Aortic valve
  B.   Pulmonic valve
  C.   Tricuspid valve
  D.   Mitral valve

Answer: A. Normally, the aortic valve closes before the pulmonic valve because the pressure is higher in the aorta. In a paradoxical S_2 split, the closing of the aortic valve is delayed.

Scoring

☆☆☆ If you answered all five questions correctly, splendid! Split heart sounds could be your specialty; you seem to know them by heart.

☆☆ If you answered four questions correctly, super! You've heard all of the information; now you can put it into practice.

☆ If you answered fewer than four questions correctly, don't split! You've got time to go back and review this chapter and go over what you missed.

S_3 and S_4 heart sounds

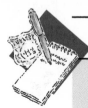

Just the facts

In this chapter, you'll learn:

♦ left ventricular diastolic filling sounds

♦ differences between S_1 and S_2 and S_3 and S_4

♦ characteristics of normal and abnormal S_3

♦ characteristics of normal and abnormal S_4.

A closer look at S_3 and S_4

The first and second heart sounds, S_1 and S_2, mark the beginning and end, respectively, of ventricular systole and associated valve closures. In healthy individuals, these two sounds and their components are relatively easy to hear during auscultation and are best heard with the diaphragm of the stethoscope.

Gotta be different

The two left ventricular diastolic filling sounds, S_3 and S_4, are sometimes heard over the mitral area. These sounds differ from S_1 and S_2 in that they're low-frequency sounds and are produced by ventricular filling rather than by valve closures.

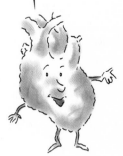

S_3 and S_4 are low-frequency sounds produced by ventricular filling.

Third heart sound, S_3

Occasionally, a physiologic S_3 is heard during auscultation after S_2. S_3 sounds are caused by vibrations occurring during rapid, passive ventricular filling. Early in diastole, after isovolumic relaxation, the mitral and tricuspid valves open and the ventricles fill and expand. (See *Understanding S_3.*)

For the young at heart

S_3 is considered normal in children and healthy individuals under age 20 as well as in very athletic young adults. In children and young adults, the left ventricle is normally compliant, permitting rapid filling. The left ventricle responds with an abrupt change in wall motion that causes a sudden decrease in blood flow. These events generate vibrations, which are responsible for physiologic S_3. The more vigorously the left ventricle expands, the greater the chances are that an S_3 will occur.

High output

A physiologic S_3 is also commonly audible in patients with high-output conditions, in which rapid ventricular expansion caused by increased blood volume is present. Anemia, fever, pregnancy, and thyrotoxicosis are some of the conditions that cause rapid ventricular expansion, resulting in an S_3.

An S_3 is also commonly heard in young, slender individuals during periods of excessive catecholamine release, such as in pheochromocytoma, acute myocardial infarction (MI), acute alcohol withdrawal, cocaine abuse, stroke, or severe heart failure. In older adults and elderly patients, an S_3 may be the first indication of heart failure.

Characteristics of S_3

S_3 is usually heard best near the apex of the heart, over the mitral area. (See *Auscultating for S_3.*)

Characteristics include:
• varying intensity and loudness (sometimes soft and faint intensity and difficult to hear; other times loud and easy to hear)
• heard best during expiration when blood flow into the left ventricle is increased **(23)** (see *Tips for hearing S_3*)
• short duration
• possibly intermittent occurrence during every third or fourth heartbeat
• dull, thudlike quality.

Understanding S_3

The third heart sound (S_3) is caused by vibration of the ventricles during ventricular filling, which occurs when the mitral and tricuspid valves open.

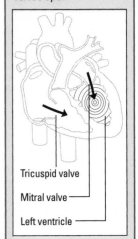

Tricuspid valve

Mitral valve

Left ventricle

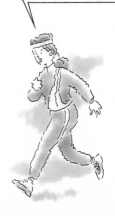

S_3 is normal in children and healthy individuals under age 20 or in very athletic young adults.

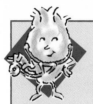

Location, location, location

Auscultating for S_3

To listen for a third heart sound (S_3), place your stethoscope over the mitral area, located in the fifth intercostal space at the mid-clavicular line (shown below).

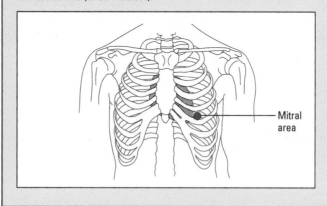

Mitral area

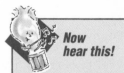

Now hear this!

Tips for hearing S_3

Here are some tips that can enhance your ability to auscultate and palpate for a third heart sound (S_3):

• Place the patient in a partial left lateral recumbent position.

• Usually, S_3 is heard best with the bell of the stethoscope over the mitral area, and it can usually be palpated over the same area.

• Because S_3 is associated with blood volume and velocity, it can be intensified by maneuvers that increase stroke volume, such as elevating the patient's legs from a recumbent position or having the patient exercise briefly or cough several times.

• S_3 commonly disappears with maneuvers that decrease venous return, such as having the patient sit up or stand.

Time after time

S_3 is heard early in diastole. Its timing is closely related to S_2, which is heard just after the T wave, and follows S_2 by 0.14 to 0.20 second. **(24)** The relationship of S_3 to the electrocardiogram (ECG) waveform can be seen easily on a phonocardiogram (PCG); on the ECG, S_3 occurs during the TP interval just after the T wave. Normally, the S_2-S_3 interval is reliably constant. (See *Physiologic S_3 on PCG and ECG*, page 80.)

Abnormal S_3

As a person ages, the heart's left ventricle becomes less compliant. Decreased ventricular compliance leads to pressure changes, which cause slowed left ventricular isovolumic relaxation and reduced blood flow velocity into the ventricle. (See *Understanding abnormal S_3*, page 80.)

Gallop

An audible S_3 that's present after age 20 is considered abnormal unless the individual is a highly trained athlete.

Physiologic S$_3$ on PCG and ECG

A third heart sound (S$_3$) usually follows a second heart sound (S$_2$) by 0.14 to 0.20 second. The timing is relatively constant between the TP intervals, as shown on the phonocardiogram (PCG) and electrocardiogram (ECG) representation below.

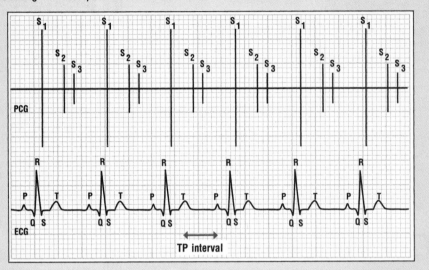

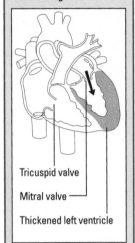

Understanding abnormal S$_3$

An abnormal third heart sound (S$_3$) occurs when the left ventricle becomes less compliant or thickened, which may occur because of increased age.

Tricuspid valve

Mitral valve

Thickened left ventricle

This abnormal S$_1$, S$_2$, S$_3$ sequence is referred to as a *ventricular gallop* or *gallop rhythm*. **(25)** An abnormal S$_3$ has the same sound characteristics, is heard over the same location (the mitral area), and has the same timing in relation to S$_2$ as a physiologic S$_3$. The differences between the two are related to the patient's age and clinical condition. Also, an S$_3$ gallop rhythm usually persists despite maneuvers that decrease venous return. **(26)**

Pump up the volume

An abnormal S$_3$ is heard in conditions associated with increased blood volume and increased inflow velocity into the left ventricle. It's heard with or without an increase in ventricular diastolic pressure. Consequently, a patient with mitral insufficiency or heart failure may have an abnormal S$_3$. This heart sound can also be heard during increased blood flow through the mitral valve, which occurs in patients

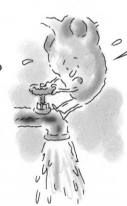

Abnormal S$_3$ can be heard in patients who have conditions associated with increased blood volume and increased inflow velocity into the left ventricle.

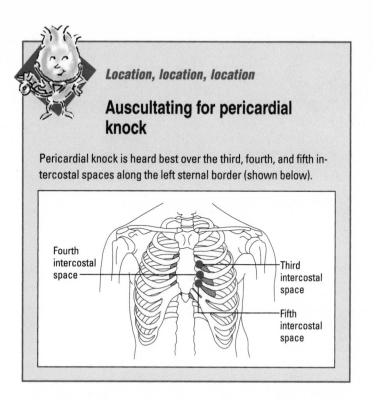

Location, location, location

Auscultating for pericardial knock

Pericardial knock is heard best over the third, fourth, and fifth intercostal spaces along the left sternal border (shown below).

Fourth intercostal space

Third intercostal space

Fifth intercostal space

with ventricular septal defects, patent ductus arteriosus, or severe aortic insufficiency.

Pericardial knock

An abnormal S$_3$ in patients with constrictive pericarditis is called *pericardial knock*. This type of abnormal S$_3$ occurs closer to S$_2$. The interval between S$_2$ and S$_3$ is usually less than 0.14 second. **(27)** With the diaphragm of the stethoscope, the pericardial knock is easier to hear than a normal or abnormal S$_3$. **(28)** Inspiration usually intensifies pericardial knock. (See *Auscultating for pericardial knock.*)

Right-sided S$_3$

Because the right ventricle is normally much more compliant than the left ventricle, its filling shouldn't cause vibrations that create an S$_3$. However, in some patients, an S$_3$ originates in the right ventricle instead of the left. When it does, it's always considered abnormal. **(29)** Right-sided S$_3$ is more prominent during inspiration because of in-

Location, location, location

Auscultating for right-sided S_3

A right-sided third heart sound (S_3) is heard best over the third, fourth, and fifth intercostal spaces and over the epigastric area.

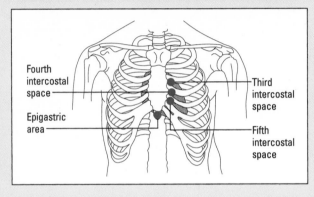

Fourth intercostal space

Epigastric area

Third intercostal space

Fifth intercostal space

Understanding right-sided S_3

It's easy to remember that a right-sided third heart sound (S_3) occurs when the right ventricle isn't compliant. Right-sided S_3 is always considered abnormal.

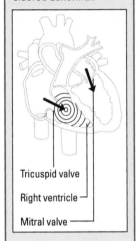

Tricuspid valve

Right ventricle

Mitral valve

creased blood flow into the right ventricle. (See *Understanding right-sided S_3*.)

Wrong on the right

Patients with enlarged right ventricles commonly have right-sided S_3. This heart sound is audible in patients with right-sided heart failure, pulmonic insufficiency, or severe tricuspid insufficiency. **(30)** (See *Auscultating for right-sided S_3*.)

Fourth heart sound, S_4

By the end of diastole, the ventricles are nearly full; atrial contraction further stretches and fills the ventricles. The vibrations caused by this stretching and filling in late diastole generate an additional heart sound, S_4, sometimes called an *atrial diastolic gallop*. **(31)** (See *Understanding S_4*.)

S_4 results from vibrations caused by the filling of the ventricles and stretching in late diastole. It's sometimes called *atrial diastolic gallop*.

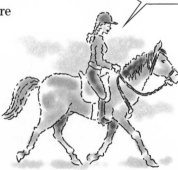

Break from the norm

An S_4 is almost always abnormal, except in highly trained young athletes with physiologic left ventricular hypertrophy. Because S_4 is associated with atrial contraction, it isn't produced in conditions in which atrial systole doesn't occur, such as atrial fibrillation.

Characteristics of S_4

S_4 is usually located near the heart's apex over the mitral area; occasionally, it's also palpable over this area. (See *Auscultating for S_4.*)

Other characteristics of S_4 include:
• varying intensity and loudness (sometimes faint intensity, making it difficult to hear; other times, loud and easily heard)
• relatively short duration and intermittent occurrence, during every third or fourth heartbeat
• low pitch that's heard best with the bell of the stethoscope
• thudlike quality
• presystolic timing

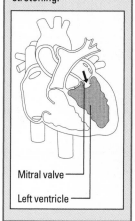

Understanding S_4

A fourth heart sound (S_4) is produced when the ventricles are filling and stretching.

Mitral valve

Left ventricle

Location, location, location

Auscultating for S_4

To best hear a fourth heart sound (S_4), place the bell of the stethoscope over the mitral area (shown below).

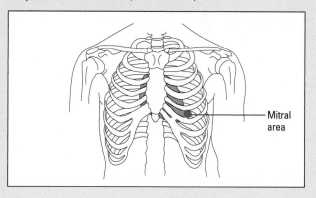

Mitral area

S$_4$ on PCG and ECG

A fourth heart sound (S$_4$) is easy to see on the phonocardiogram (PCG) and electrocardiogram (ECG) representation below. S$_4$ occurs before the first heart sound (S$_1$) during the PR interval.

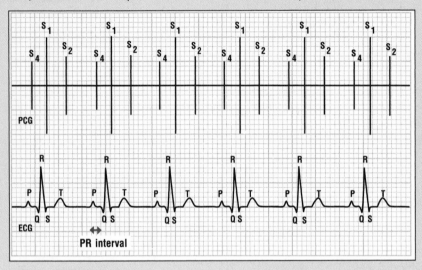

- relationship to S$_1$ easily seen in the ECG waveform
- occurrence during PR interval and before S$_1$ **(32)** (see *S$_4$ on PCG and ECG*).

Abnormal S$_4$

An abnormal S$_4$ is almost always associated with increased mean left atrial pressure caused by a noncompliant left ventricle. It's heard during or after an acute MI as well as in patients with:

- hypertension (the most common cause)
- cardiomyopathies, especially hypertrophic cardiomyopathy
- ischemic heart disease.

When S$_4$ is heard in a patient with hypertension, systolic blood pressure usually exceeds 160 mm Hg or diastolic pressure exceeds 100 mm Hg.

Oh no, overload

An abnormal S$_4$ can also accompany certain volume overload conditions, such as:

> When S$_4$ is heard in a patient with hypertension, systolic blood pressure usually exceeds 160 mm Hg or diastolic pressure exceeds 100 mm Hg.

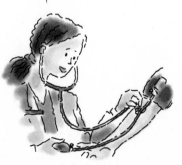

- hyperthyroidism
- certain anemias
- sudden severe mitral insufficiency.

Summation gallop

Normally, S$_4$ precedes S$_1$ by an appreciable interval that correlates with the PR interval on the ECG. However, in patients with first-degree atrioventricular block, the P wave occurs early in diastole and S$_4$ may occur during the early rapid diastolic filling period.

Likewise, in tachycardia, S$_4$ may cover up S$_3$ during early rapid filling. If either of these conditions exists, the S$_4$ fuses with S$_3$ to become a single diastolic filling sound called a *summation gallop*, which may be louder than S$_4$, S$_3$, or S$_1$. **(33)** (See *Summation gallop on PCG and ECG*.)

Summation gallop on PCG and ECG

In summation gallop, a fourth heart sound (S$_4$) may occur early or cover up the third heart sound (S$_3$), thus becoming a single diastolic filling sound. Summation gallop may be louder than S$_4$, S$_3$, and the first heart sound (S$_1$). This pattern is shown on the phonocardiogram (PCG) and electrocardiogram (ECG) representation below.

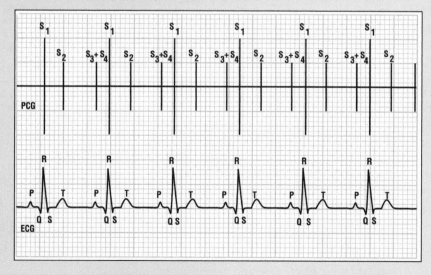

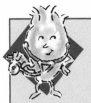

Location, location, location

Auscultating for right-sided S₄

A right-sided fourth heart sound (S₄) is heard best over the third, fourth, and fifth intercostal spaces along the left sternal border and over the epigastric area (shown below) with the patient in a supine position.

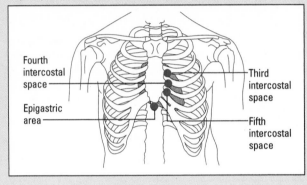

Fourth intercostal space

Epigastric area

Third intercostal space

Fifth intercostal space

Understanding right-sided S₄

A right-sided fourth heart sound (S₄) occurs when S₄ occurs in the right ventricle instead of the left, as shown below.

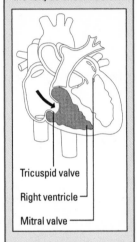

Tricuspid valve

Right ventricle

Mitral valve

Right-sided S₄

S_4 generated in the right ventricle is called a *right-sided S_4.* **(34)** (See *Understanding right-sided S_4.*) It's commonly heard in conditions that increase pressure in the right ventricle by more than 100 mm Hg, such as pulmonic stenosis or pulmonary hypertension. Although the sound may vary with respiration, it's more audible during inspiration. (See *Auscultating for right-sided S_4.*)

S_4 is commonly heard in such conditions as pulmonic stenosis and pulmonary hypertension.

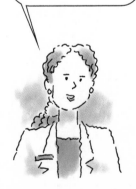

Differentiating S₄ from S₁ split

Distinguishing an S_1 split (M_1-T_1) from an S_4-S_1 sequence is sometimes difficult. Here are some tips to help you distinguish them:

• An S_1 split is heard best between the mitral and tricuspid areas with the diaphragm of the stethoscope, whereas an S_4 is heard best over the mitral area with the bell of the stethoscope and usually isn't audible with the diaphragm. (See *Tips for hearing S_4.*)

• An S_4 may be palpable.

• An S_1 split is a systolic ejection sound, which is higher in pitch than S_4.

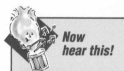

S₃ and S₄: Similarities and differences

S_3, like S_4, is low-pitched and may be faint or loud and heard only intermittently. Both sounds are heard best at the heart's apex, located over the mitral area, using the bell of the stethoscope, with the patient in a partial left lateral recumbent position. Both sounds vary with respirations and can be enhanced by maneuvers that increase stroke volume, such as elevating the patient's legs while in a recumbent position or having him perform handgrip exercises.

Just remember this

At times, differentiating S_3 from S_4 is difficult. Remember that S_3 is heard after S_2, whereas S_4 occurs at the beginning of atrial systole and therefore occurs before S_1.

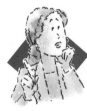

Quick quiz

1. S_1 and S_2 differ from S_3 and S_4 because S_1 and S_2 are produced by:
  A.   valves closing.
  B.   ventricular filling.
  C.   atrial filling.
  D.   low-pitched sounds.

Answer: A. S_1 and S_2 sounds are produced by valve closure and have high-pitched sounds. S_3 and S_4 are produced by the vibrations from ventricular filling and produce low-pitched sounds.

2. Which of the following conditions is commonly associated with S_3?
  A.   Hypertension
  B.   Asthma
  C.   Thyrotoxicosis
  D.   Diabetes

Answer: C. S_3 occurs in patients with high-output conditions in which rapid ventricular expansion and increased blood volume is present, including anemia, fever, thyrotoxicosis, and pregnancy. S_3 is also common in children and young, thin, athletic adults.

Tips for hearing S₄

To enhance your auscultation for the fourth heart sound (S_4), place the patient in the partial left lateral recumbent position, which brings the heart closer to the chest wall. To increase the intensity of S_4, have the patient perform maneuvers that increase left atrial pressure, such as handgrip exercises.

3.   A physiologic S$_3$ has the same sound characteristics as:
  A.   S$_4$.
  B.   abnormal S$_4$.
  C.   abnormal S$_3$.
  D.   right-sided S$_3$.

Answer: C. A physiologic S$_3$ has the same sound characteristics as an abnormal S$_3$. The differences between these two sounds are related to the patient's age and clinical condition.

4.   In which of the following areas should you listen to best hear an S$_4$?
  A.   Mitral
  B.   Tricuspid
  C.   Aortic
  D.   Pulmonic

Answer: A. To best hear an S$_4$, place the bell of the stethoscope over the mitral area.

5.   An S$_4$ that occurs during early rapid diastolic filling is referred to as:
  A.   an atrial diastolic gallop.
  B.   a summation gallop.
  C.   a right-sided S$_4$.
  D.   pericardial knock.

Answer: B. When a P wave occurs early in diastole, S$_4$ may occur during the early rapid diastolic filling period and superimpose itself on S$_3$, thus fusing together and producing a single diastolic filling sound known as a *summation gallop*.

Scoring

☆☆☆ If you answered all five questions correctly, terrific! Your summation of this chapter is superb. Gallop on to the next chapter.

☆☆ If you answered four questions correctly, you're pumping away at these questions with all of your heart! Keep up the good work.

☆ If you answered fewer than four questions correctly, you've still got a lot of heart! Split the chapter in halves and review it again.

Other diastolic and systolic sounds

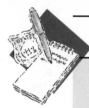

Just the facts

In this chapter, you'll learn:

♦ characteristics of opening snaps

♦ characteristics of systolic ejection sounds

♦ characteristics of midsystolic clicks

♦ differentiation of these other diastolic and systolic sounds from other heart sounds.

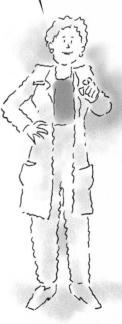

> You've learned about S_1, S_2, S_3, and S_4. Now it's time for opening snaps, systolic ejection sounds, and midsystolic clicks.

Understanding other diastolic and systolic sounds

In previous chapters, you've learned about several different types of heart sounds, including S_1, S_2, S_3, and S_4. However, other systolic and diastolic sounds exist as well, such as opening snap, systolic ejection sound, and midsystolic click.

Opening snap

At the end of ventricular systole, the aortic and pulmonic valves close, generating the second heart sound (S_2). S_2 is followed by a brief period of isovolumic relaxation; during this time, ventricular pressure falls. When ventricular pressure is less than atrial pressure, the mitral and tricuspid valves open. In a healthy heart, the mitral and tricuspid valves open silently during diastole. In certain pathologic states, these atrioventricular valves will open more rapidly than normal and make a sound known as an *opening snap* (OS). This snap sound is caused when valve leaflets become stenotic or abnormally narrowed (such as in patients with a history of rheumatic fever) while remaining somewhat mobile. **(35)** (See *Understanding an OS.*)

Might be mitral

Causes of mitral valve OS include:
- mitral stenosis (most common)
- mitral stenosis with a mobile valve
- rapid mitral flow, which causes a soft snap (such as left-to-right shunt in ventricular septal defect or patent ductus arteriosus)
- severe mitral insufficiency.

Rare but snappy

A tricuspid OS is rare and may be caused by:
- tricuspid valve abnormalities (such as rheumatic stenosis)
- increased tricuspid flow (such as left-to-right shunt in an atrial septal defect).

Sounds like murmur to me

An OS is generated by the maximum opening of the leaflets, which is somewhat limited because of stenosis. The OS usually indicates the beginning of a diastolic murmur associated with mitral stenosis. The intensity of the OS is directly proportional to the motility of the valve and the degree of fusion of the valve's cusps. The timing of the OS is influenced by atrial pressure (higher pressure equals earlier snap) and the duration of the isovolumetric relaxation phase (shorter relaxation phase equals earlier OS). If the mitral valve becomes severely calcified and inflexible, the OS disappears.

Understanding an OS

An opening snap (OS) is caused by stenotic, yet mobile, mitral valve leaflets. The location of these leaflets is shown below.

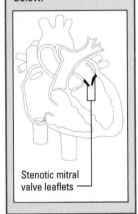

Stenotic mitral valve leaflets —

Characteristics of an OS

An OS is usually heard best near the heart's apex over the mitral area or just medial to it. (See *Auscultating for an OS.*) Its intensity varies among patients; however, it's usually easy to hear during auscultation. To distinguish the OS from P_2, auscultate for the heart sounds during inspiration to hear A_2, P_2, and the OS in quick succession.

Other sound characteristics include:
- short duration
- high pitch that's heard best with the diaphragm of the stethoscope

Auscultating for an OS

An opening snap (OS) is heard best with the diaphragm of the stethoscope near the heart's apex over the mitral area (shown below) or just medial to it. An OS is also transmitted widely across the precordium and can usually be heard over the aortic, pulmonic, and tricuspid areas.

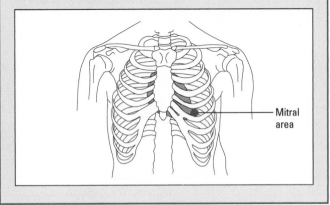

Mitral area

An OS has several distinguishing characteristics, and it's usually heard best near the heart's apex over the mitral area.

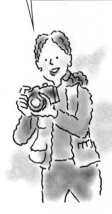

- distinctive sharp, crisp, snaplike quality
- higher pitch than S_2
- as loud as or louder than S_2
- timing closely related to S_2
- occurrence early in ventricular diastole, just after the stenotic mitral valve opens
- occurrence just after the T wave in the electrocardiogram (ECG) waveform. **(36)** (See *OS on PCG and ECG*, page 92.)

Differentiating OS from S_2

An OS occurs early in diastole and consequently may be confused with the pulmonic component (P_2) or S_3. One characteristic of an OS that helps distinguish it from P_2 is its timing: The aortic component (A_2)-P_2 interval is normally shorter than the A_2-OS interval. Also, when the patient stands, the A_2-P_2 interval narrows, whereas the A_2-OS interval widens.

OS on PCG and ECG

An opening snap (OS) is heard closely after the second heart sound (S_2), just after the T wave, as shown on the phonocardiogram (PCG) and electrocardiogram (ECG) representation below.

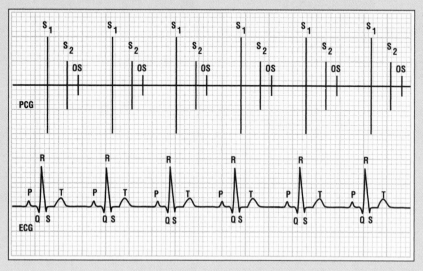

Another characteristic is that the A_2-OS interval remains constant throughout respiration, whereas the A_2-P_2 interval normally widens during inspiration and narrows during expiration. During inspiration, three distinct sounds can usually be heard over the pulmonic area; therefore, the sequence must be A_2, P_2, OS. In contrast, during expiration, the A_2-P_2 interval narrows or fuses, forming one sound. This creates an S_2-OS interval.

I overheard...

Finally, P_2 isn't usually heard over the mitral area. Therefore, if you hear a split S_2 over this area, it may be an S_2 and an OS.

The sound difference between an OS and an S_2 is simple. Three distinct sounds can usually be heard: A_2, P_2, and OS.

Well, the sound difference between OS and S_3 is a bit more complicated. Timing can help to distinguish the difference.

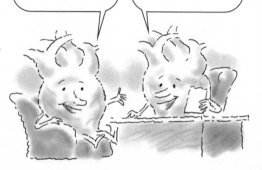

Differentiating OS from S_3

Distinguishing an OS from an S_3 is difficult in some patients, especially in those with mild mitral stenosis when the A_2-OS interval is wider than usual and the OS is somewhat softer. One characteristic of an OS that helps distinguish it from an S_3 is its timing. Also, the A_2-S_3 interval is usually longer than the A_2-OS interval. Furthermore, S_3 is a low-frequency sound that's heard best over the mitral area with the bell of the stethoscope. In contrast, an OS produces a high-frequency sound that's more widely transmitted across the precordium and is heard best with the diaphragm.

Intense OS

Another characteristic of an OS is that its intensity usually isn't affected by having the patient stand, whereas S_3 intensity can be increased by increasing stroke volume through such activities as standing, coughing, or exercising briefly. Finally, if the murmur typically heard in patients with mitral stenosis is present, you can confirm that the sound is an OS. (See *Tips for hearing an OS*.)

Now hear this!

Tips for hearing an OS

When auscultating for an opening snap (OS) of the mitral valve, know that it has a quality similar to a normal heart sound and is commonly confused with a splitting S_2. The brief, sharp, snapping sound is heard shortly after the aortic component (A_2) of S_2.

Stethoscope for snap
To hear an OS better, place the stethoscope midway between the pulmonic and mitral areas. When loud, it's widely transmitted over the entire precordium. In addition, turn the patient to the left lateral position because standing tends to lower left atrial pressure and thus increase the A_2-OS interval.

Exercise intensifies
Remember that a soft OS may be intensified after exercise, which increases atrial pressure. Although the A_2-OS interval isn't altered during different phases of respiration, the mitral valve OS is usually heard loudest on expiration.

Systolic ejection sound

Just as an OS is caused by stenotic mitral valve leaflets, a systolic ejection sound (SES) is caused by the opening of a stenotic aortic or pulmonic valve. Systolic ejection murmurs are discussed in depth in chapter 9; however, here's a short overview on SESs.

In brief

An SES usually occurs early in systole after S_1 and isovolumic contraction. It's commonly associated with ventricular ejection and the maximum opening of a stenotic, yet mobile, aortic or pulmonic valve. If the valve is severely stenotic because of calcification, an SES—like an OS—won't be produced. (See *Understanding an SES*.)

It's abnormal all right...

An SES is considered an abnormal condition whether it originates in the heart's right or left side. It may also be caused by sudden distention of an already dilated aorta or pulmonary artery and by forceful ventricular ejection from pulmonary or systemic hypertension.

Pulmonic ejection sound

A pulmonic ejection sound (PES) is the only right-sided heart sound that increases in intensity during expiration and diminishes or disappears during inspiration. **(37)**

Sounds of respiration

In a normal heart, inspiration increases right ventricular volume, causing the pulmonic leaflet valve to form a dome shape toward the pulmonary artery, which decreases the sound's intensity. During expiration, right ventricular volume is decreased, the valve leaflet is less domed, and its opening produces a louder snap. In a patient with pulmonary artery dilation or pulmonary hypertension, a PES may not vary in intensity during respiration.

PES presence

Because a PES may occur in idiopathic dilation of the pulmonary artery but usually isn't present in supravalvular or muscular subvalvular obstructions, its presence can be

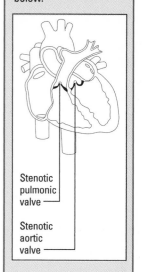

Understanding an SES

A systolic ejection sound (SES) is produced from a stenotic, yet mobile, aortic or pulmonic valve. The locations of these valves are shown below.

Stenotic pulmonic valve —

Stenotic aortic valve —

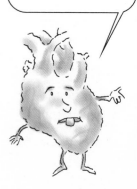

An SES is an abnormal condition — whether it originates from my right or left side.

used to differentiate between these conditions. Occasionally, a PES may also be heard with atrial and ventricular septal defects.

Characteristics of a PES

A PES is usually heard best near the heart's base over the pulmonic area. (See *Auscultating for a PES.*)

Other sound characteristics include:
- soft intensity (may be equal to or greater than that of S_1)
- short duration
- a high pitch that's heard best with the diaphragm of the stethoscope
- a sharp or clicklike quality
- timing that's closely related to S_1 (see *Differentiating PES and S_1*)
- occurrence early in ventricular systole, just after the opening of a stenotic pulmonic valve **(38)**
- occurrence just after the QRS complex (see *PES on PCG and ECG*, page 96).

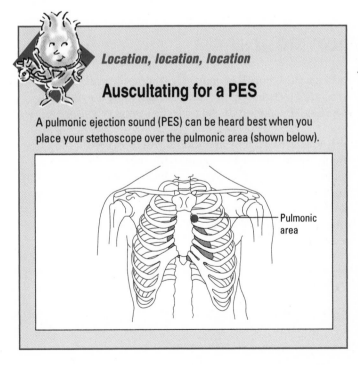

Location, location, location

Auscultating for a PES

A pulmonic ejection sound (PES) can be heard best when you place your stethoscope over the pulmonic area (shown below).

Pulmonic area

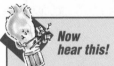

Now hear this!

Differentiating PES and S_1

To differentiate between a pulmonic ejection sound (PES) and first heart sound (S_1), remember that a PES is heard in the pulmonic area and varies with respiration. A split S_1 is heard in the tricuspid area and doesn't vary with respiration.

PES on PCG and ECG

A pulmonic ejection sound (PES) is closely related to the first heart sound (S_1). It occurs just after S_1, after the QRS complex, as shown on the phonocardiogram (PCG) and electrocardiogram (ECG) representation below.

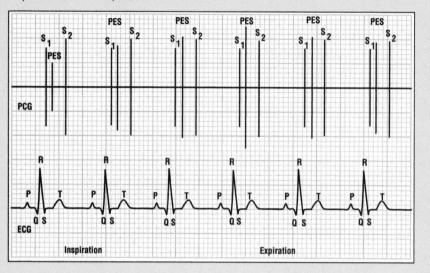

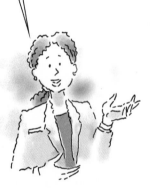

Unlike a PES, which is caused by pulmonic valve stenosis, an AES is caused by aortic valve stenosis.

Aortic ejection sound

Unlike a PES, which is caused by pulmonic valve stenosis, an aortic ejection sound (AES) is caused by aortic valve stenosis. This sound doesn't vary in intensity with respiration.

An AES may occur in patients with aortic root dilation, which is commonly associated with such conditions as systemic hypertension, an ascending aortic aneurysm, or coarctation of the aorta. An AES may also be heard in patients with aortic stenosis or aortic insufficiency, but the sound is less clicklike when it's associated with aortic insufficiency. **(39)**

Characteristics of an AES

An AES is heard best near the heart's apex over the mitral area, near the heart's base over the aortic area, or over Erb's point. (See *Auscultating for an AES.*)

Memory jogger

To remember the causes of **PES** and **AES**, think:

PVS (pulmonic valve stenosis) causes **PES**

AVS (aortic valve stenosis) causes **AES**.

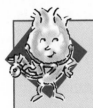

Auscultating for an AES

An aortic ejection sound (AES) is high in pitch. To listen for an AES, place your stethoscope over any of the areas identified below.

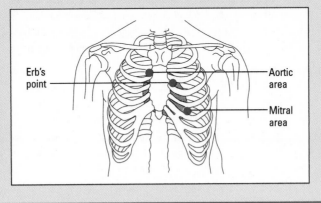

Other sound characteristics include:
- soft intensity (may be equal to or greater than that of S_1)
- short duration
- high pitch that's heard best with the diaphragm of the stethoscope
- sharp or clicklike quality
- timing that's closely related to S_1 **(40)** (see *Differentiating AES from other heart sounds*, page 98)
- occurrence early in ventricular systole, just after the opening of a stenotic aortic valve
- occurrence just after the QRS complex in the ECG waveform.

Midsystolic click

A midsystolic click (MSC) occurs when the prolapsed mitral valve's leaflets and chordae tendineae become tense. The anterior or posterior leaflet, or both leaflets, can prolapse. Occasionally, multiple clicks occur that are heard in midsystole to late systole; they're heard best over the tricuspid area and toward the mitral area. Like an ejection

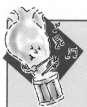

Now hear this!

Differentiating AES from other heart sounds

Certain characteristics help to distinguish an aortic ejection sound (AES) from other heart sounds. One such characteristic is that an AES radiates more than a pulmonic ejection sound. Another characteristic is that a split first heart sound heard over the mitral area is more likely to be a mitral component than an AES.

Remember this
You can differentiate an AES from a fourth heart sound (S4) by remembering that S4 is heard best with the bell of the stethoscope over the mitral area and is usually accompanied by a palpable, presystolic apical bulge. Also, an S4 is intensified by maneuvers that increase left atrial pressure, such as brief exercise, squatting, or coughing. An AES isn't affected by any of these maneuvers.

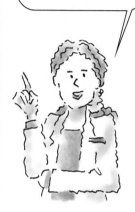

Keep in mind that, like an ES, a midsystolic to late-systolic click is a crisp, high-frequency sound.

sound (ES), these midsystolic to late-systolic clicks are crisp, high-frequency sounds. **(41)** (See *Understanding an MSC.*)

Characteristics of an MSC

An MSC is usually heard best over the tricuspid area and near the heart's apex over the mitral area. (See *Auscultating for an MSC.*)

Other characteristics include:
• intensity equal to or greater than that of S_1
• short duration
• high pitch that's heard best with the diaphragm of the stethoscope
• clicklike quality
• variability of the click's timing, occurring in early systole, midsystole, or late systole
• occurrence during the QT interval on the ECG waveform **(42)** (see *MSC on PCG and ECG*, page 100).

Understanding an MSC

Midsystolic click (MSC) occurs when the anterior or posterior mitral valve leaflets prolapse and the chordae tendineae tense, as shown below.

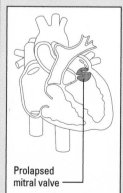

Prolapsed mitral valve

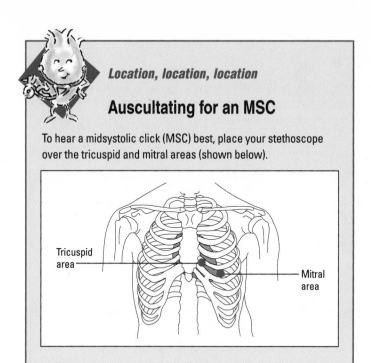

Location, location, location

Auscultating for an MSC

To hear a midsystolic click (MSC) best, place your stethoscope over the tricuspid and mitral areas (shown below).

Tricuspid area

Mitral area

Moving in time

The timing of an MSC is affected by various movements, such as having the patient stand or performing Valsalva's maneuver. Such maneuvers result in reduced left ventricular filling and cause the MSC to be heard closer to S_1. The MSC may even merge with S_1 or disappear completely. Increasing left ventricular volume by raising the legs from a recumbent position or squatting delays the click. This maneuver may also cause the prolapse not to occur and the MSC to be diminished or inaudible.

Accompanying tunes

Sometimes an MSC is accompanied by a late systolic crescendo murmur or the characteristic holosystolic murmur of mitral insufficiency. An MSC may also be caused by such extracardiac conditions as pleuropericardial adhesions, atrial septal aneurysms, and cardiac tumors.

An MSC can be caused by such extracardiac conditions as pleuropericardial adhesions, atrial septal aneurysms, and cardiac tumors.

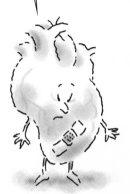

MSC on PCG and ECG

Note that a midsystolic click (MCS) occurs during the QT interval, as shown on the phonocardiogram (PCG) and electrocardiogram (ECG) representation below.

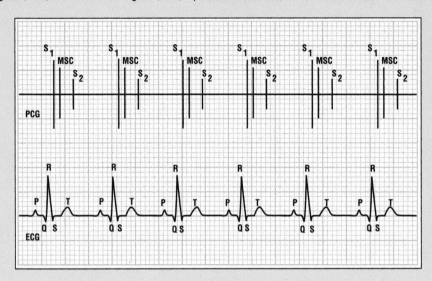

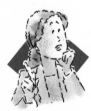

Quick quiz

1. An OS is caused by a:
   A.   stenosed aortic valve.
   B.   stenosed tricuspid valve.
   C.   stenosed mitral valve.
   D.   stenosed pulmonic valve.

Answer: C. OS occurs when the mitral valve leaflets become stenosed or abnormally narrowed but remain somewhat mobile, such as in patients with a history of rheumatic fever.

2. To differentiate an OS from an S_2, remember that the:
    A. A_2-OS interval is shorter than the A_2-P_2 interval.
    B. A_2-OS interval narrows when the patient stands.
    C. A_2-OS interval stays constant during respiration.
    D. A_2-OS interval narrows during expiration.

Answer: C. Unlike the A_2-P_2 interval, the A_2-OS interval is longer than the A_2-P_2 interval. Also, the A_2-OS interval widens when the patient stands but remains constant during respiration.

3. While auscultating a patient, you hear an SES. You know that an SES is caused by a:
    A.   severely stenotic, immobile tricuspid or mitral valve.
    B.   stenotic, yet mobile, tricuspid or mitral valve.
    C.   severely stenotic, immobile aortic or pulmonic valve.
    D.   stenotic, yet mobile, aortic or pulmonic valve.

Answer: D. An SES is caused by a stenotic, yet mobile, aortic or pulmonic valve. Similar to an OS, no sound is produced when the valve is severely stenotic and immobile.

4. To differentiate an AES from a PES, you should remember that:
    A.   AES increases in intensity during inspiration.
    B.   PES increases in intensity during expiration.
    C.   AES decreases in intensity during inspiration.
    D.   PES decreases in intensity during expiration.

Answer: B. PES is the only right-sided heart sound that increases in intensity during expiration and disappears during inspiration. AES doesn't vary in intensity during inspiration or expiration.

5. To better hear an MSC, auscultate:
    A.   the entire precordial area.
    B.   the pulmonic area.
    C.   Erb's point
    D.   the tricuspid area.

Answer: D. An MSC is usually heard best over the tricuspid area and near the heart's apex over the mitral area.

6. An MSC may be caused by extracardiac conditions. One example of an extracardiac cause is:

    A.   thoracic aortic aneurysm.

    B.   pleuropericardial adhesions.

    C.   esophageal diverticula.

    D.   polymyositis.

Answer. B. Pleuropericardial adhesions, as well as atrial septal aneurysms and cardiac tumors, are extracardiac causes of MSC.

Scoring

☆☆☆ If you answered all six questions correctly, outstanding! When it comes to understanding other diastolic and systolic sounds, your heart is in the right place.

☆☆ If you answered four or five questions correctly, great job! The information has obviously clicked for you.

☆ If you answered fewer than four questions correctly, snap out of it! It's time to take a breather and review this chapter one more time.

Murmur fundamentals

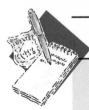

Just the facts

In this chapter, you'll learn:

♦ the process by which turbulent blood flow produces murmurs

♦ seven characteristics used to describe murmurs

♦ murmur grading, using the six-point graded scale

♦ the proper way to explain a murmur's configuration.

A look at murmurs

A murmur is an abnormal, usually periodic sound of short duration that's heard during auscultation. A murmur may be benign or may be caused by a medical condition. Many different types of murmurs exist; specific murmur types are discussed in later chapters.

Causes

Whereas heart sounds are produced by brief vibrations that correspond to the beginning and end of systole, murmurs are produced by a prolonged series of vibrations that occur during systole and diastole. These vibrations result from turbulent blood flow.

Murmuring brook

Longer than a heart sound, a murmur occurs as a vibrating, blowing, or rumbling noise. Just as water in a stream "babbles" as it passes through a narrow point, turbulent blood flow produces a murmur.

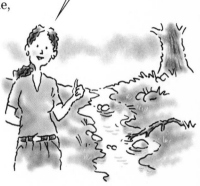

The sound of a heart murmur is a lot like the sound of a babbling brook.

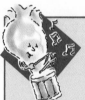

Now hear this!

Tips for listening to murmurs

Here are some tips that can help improve your murmur auscultation:

• Initially, learn to identify the loudest location and pinpoint the timing of murmurs.

• As your auscultation techniques improve, try to identify the intensity, duration, pitch, quality, and configuration.

• The best way to hear murmurs is with the patient sitting up and leaning forward. You can also ask the patient to lie on his left side.

Turbulence ahead

Several conditions—such as blood flowing at a high velocity through a partially obstructed opening, blood flowing from a higher pressure chamber to a lower pressure one, or any combination of these—can cause turbulent blood flow. Other causes of turbulence include structural defects in the heart's chambers or valves and changes in the viscosity of the blood or the speed of blood flow. You may hear these heart murmurs over the same precordial areas during auscultation. (See *Tips for listening to murmurs.*)

Murmur characteristics

Murmurs, like other heart sounds, are described by several audible characteristics that are heard during auscultation. The terms used to describe a specific characteristic are determined primarily by the volume and speed of blood flow as blood moves through the heart.

Super seven

Murmurs must be described carefully and accurately to enable easy recognition of changes in a patient's murmur characteristics and immediate assessment of the possible source of those changes. Seven characteristics are used to describe murmurs:

• location

The volume and speed of blood flow as blood moves through the heart determine specific murmur characteristics.

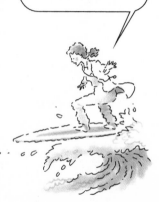

- intensity
- duration
- pitch
- quality
- timing
- configuration.

Location

A murmur's *location* is the anatomic area on the chest wall where the murmur is heard best, usually also the murmur's point of maximum intensity. This area typically correlates with the underlying location of the valve that's responsible for producing the murmur. For example, an aortic stenosis murmur is usually heard best near the heart's base over the aortic area, whereas a mitral insufficiency murmur is usually heard best near the heart's apex over the mitral area.

How radiant!

The murmur's sounds may also be transmitted to the chamber or vessel where the turbulent blood flow occurs. This phenomenon, known as *radiation*, occurs because the direction of blood flow determines sound transmission. Murmurs radiate in either a forward or a backward direction (to the neck or axillae).

Intensity

The second characteristic, *intensity*, refers to the murmur's loudness. Intensity is influenced by a patient's body weight and certain other conditions. For example, because heart sounds are affected by chest wall thickness and by certain diseases, heart sounds and murmurs are usually louder in thin individuals and fainter in obese individuals. They're also fainter in patients with emphysema, an abnormal condition of lung tissue swelling caused by the accumulation of air usually from the loss of elasticity or alveoli injury.

Hyperdynamic states, decreased blood viscosity, increased pressure gradients across valves, increased blood flow, and faster heart rates may also increase a murmur's intensity. Murmurs are less intense in hypodynamic states and in patients with an elevated hematocrit.

Grading murmurs

Use the Levine grading scale outlined below to describe a murmur's intensity:

• Grade I murmur is faint, may be heard intermittently, and is barely heard through the stethoscope.

• Grade II murmur is also audible but is quiet and soft; it's usually heard as soon as the stethoscope is placed on the chest wall.

• Grade III murmur is easily heard and is described as moderately loud.

• Grade IV murmur is loud and is usually associated with a palpable vibration known as a *thrill* or *thrust*. It also may radiate in the direction of blood flow.

• Grade V murmur is loud enough to be heard with only an edge of the stethoscope touching the chest wall; it's almost always accompanied by a palpable thrill and radiation.

• Grade VI murmur is so loud that it can be heard with the stethoscope close to, but not touching, the chest wall; it's always accompanied by a palpable thrill, and it radiates to distant structures.

Writing it down

When you document a murmur's grade, use Roman numerals as part of a fraction with VI always listed as the denominator—for example, III/VI. This means you consider the murmur to be a grade III and have used the six-point scale for assessment. That way, all health care professionals will understand which scale was used, even if they don't use the same one.

Getting the grade

Document a murmur's intensity using a uniform method. Most health care professionals use a six-point graded scale known as the Levine grading scale, with I being the faintest intensity and VI being the loudest. (See *Grading murmurs*.)

Duration

Duration is the length of time the murmur is heard during systole or diastole. It can be described as long or short.

Pitch

A murmur's *pitch*, or frequency, can vary from high to medium to low. It's usually higher in conditions accompanied by increased blood flow velocity or increased pressure gradients and lower in conditions associated with lower blood flow velocity.

Memory jogger

Want an easy way to remember that you should use a six-point scale when grading murmurs? Remember that "murmur" has six letters.

Quality

A murmur's *quality* is determined by the combination of frequencies that produces the sound. Words to describe quality may include "harsh," "rough," "musical," "scratchy," "squeaky," "rumbling," or "blowing."

Murmurs are classified by their timing in the cardiac cycle.

Timing

A murmur's *timing* refers to when the murmur occurs in the cardiac cycle. This means that the onset, duration, and end of the murmur are described in relation to systole and diastole. The beginning of systole, or S_1, can be identified easily by palpating the carotid pulse or by looking for the QRS complex on the electrocardiogram (ECG) monitor's oscilloscope.

All systolic murmurs occur between S_1 and S_2 during ventricular systole; this is the interval between the QRS complex and the T wave on the ECG waveform. All diastolic murmurs occur between S_2 and S_1 during ventricular diastole; this is the interval between the T wave and the subsequent QRS complex on the ECG waveform.

Extra class

Murmurs are further classified according to their timing within the phases of the cardiac cycle. For example, a murmur can be described as "holosystolic," meaning it's present throughout systole, or as "early systolic," "midsystolic," or "late systolic" or "diastolic."

Configuration

The last murmur characteristic, *configuration*, refers to the shape or pattern of a murmur's sound as recorded on a phonocardiogram (PCG). The configuration is usually defined by changes in the murmur's intensity during systole or diastole and is determined by blood flow pressure gradients. For example:

• A *crescendo murmur* gradually increases in intensity as the pressure gradient increases.

• A *decrescendo murmur* gradually decreases in intensity as the pressure gradient decreases.

Murmur configurations

Configurations, or patterns, refer to changes in murmur intensity.

Crescendo

A crescendo murmur becomes progressively louder.

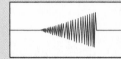

Decrescendo

A decrescendo murmur be-comes progressively softer.

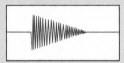

Crescendo-decrescendo

A crescendo-decrescendo murmur (also called *diamond-shaped hair*) peaks in intensity and then decreases again.

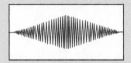

Plateau-shaped

A plateau-shaped murmur re-mains equal in intensity.

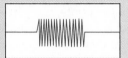

• A *crescendo-decrescendo murmur* first increases in intensity as the pressure gradient increases, then decreases in intensity as the pressure gradient decreases; it's also known as a *diamond-shaped murmur*.

• A *plateau-shaped murmur* remains equal in intensity throughout the murmur. (See *Murmur configurations*.)

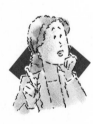

Quick quiz

1. Murmurs are caused by:
    A. brief vibrations corresponding with the beginning of systole.
    B. brief vibrations corresponding with the end of systole.
    C. closing of the aortic and pulmonic valves.
    D. a series of prolonged vibrations occurring during systole, diastole, or both due to turbulent blood flow.

Answer: D. Murmurs are caused by a series of prolonged vibrations due to turbulent blood flow.

2.   Radiation of a murmur refers to:
      A.   loudness of the murmur's sound.
      B.   timing of the murmur during the cardiac cycle.
      C.   length of time the murmur is heard during systole or diastole.
      D.   sounds transmitted to the chamber or vessel where the turbulent blood flow occurs.

Answer: D. Radiation is a phenomenon that refers to the sounds transmitted to the chamber or vessel where the turbulent blood flow occurs. It occurs because the direction of blood flow determines sound transmission.

3.   You're reading your patient's chart and find a murmur grading of III/VI. You know that this means that the patient's murmur was:
      A.   faint.
      B.   easily heard and moderately loud.
      C.   loud.
      D.   loud enough to be heard with only the edge of the stethoscope touching the chest wall and probably accompanied by a thrill and radiation.

Answer: B. Grade III murmurs on the six-point scale refer to murmurs that are easily heard and are described as moderately loud.

4.   *Configuration* refers to the:
      A.   shape or pattern of a murmur's sound.
      B.   timing of a murmur during the cardiac cycle.
      C.   length of time a murmur is heard during systole or diastole.
      D.   sounds transmitted to the chamber or vessel where the turbulent blood flow occurs.

Answer: A. Configuration is the shape or pattern of a murmur's sound as recorded on a PCG. It's defined by changes in the murmur's intensity and is determined by blood flow pressure gradients.

5. Your patient's murmur first increases in intensity but then decreases. The configuration you would use to describe this murmur is:

    A.   crescendo.
    B.   decrescendo.
    C.   diamond-shaped.
    D.   plateau-shaped.

Answer: C. A diamond-shaped murmur is also known as a *crescendo-decrescendo murmur.* This type of murmur increases in intensity as the pressure gradient increases but then decreases in intensity as the pressure gradient decreases.

Scoring

☆☆☆ If you answered all five questions correctly, congratulations! You're on your way to becoming a master of murmurs.

☆☆ If you answered four questions correctly, take heart! You've shown incredible gradient under pressure.

☆ If you answered fewer than four questions correctly, don't stop the flow! Understanding this chapter may take some time. Go back and review it.

Systolic murmurs

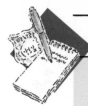

Just the facts

In this chapter, you'll learn:

♦ the way in which systolic murmurs are produced

♦ characterization of systolic murmurs

♦ different types of systolic ejection murmurs

♦ different types of systolic insufficiency murmurs.

A closer look at systolic murmurs

In a normally functioning heart, as ventricular pressures rise at the beginning of systole, the mitral and tricuspid valves close. Then, for a brief time during isovolumic contraction, while the aortic and pulmonic valves are still closed, ventricular pressures rise sharply. When the pressure in both ventricles is high enough, the aortic and pulmonic valves open and blood is ejected from the ventricles into the aorta and the pulmonary artery. Normally functioning valves facilitate this unidirectional blood flow.

Defect effects

Systolic murmurs can occur when these valves have a defect. All systolic murmurs occur during ventricular systole between the first heart sound (S_1) and the second heart sound (S_2). Aortic or pulmonic outlet abnormalities may generate forward systolic ejection murmurs (SEMs). When the mitral or tricuspid valve is involved, backward (or regurgitant) murmurs may occur. (See *Tips for hearing systolic murmurs*, page 112.)

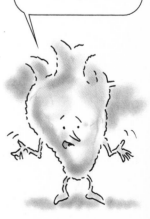

All systolic murmurs occur during ventricular systole in the presence of a defect in the mitral and tricuspid valves.

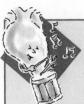

Now hear this!

Tips for hearing systolic murmurs

Usually, a systolic murmur is high-pitched (representing the high pressure and high velocity of blood during ventricular ejection); therefore, it's heard best using the diaphragm of the stethoscope.

Innocent systolic murmurs

During ventricular systole, the rapid ejection of blood from the ventricles causes turbulent blood flow that can produce innocent systolic murmurs. **(43)** These murmurs, which can be described as *benign* or *functional*, are considered normal in most patients. They can be caused simply by normal physiologic conditions, such as pregnancy, which requires a high volume of blood circulating throughout the body.

Quite commonly, innocent murmurs (also called *Still's murmurs*) can also be heard in infants or children and in thin-chested individuals. These murmurs aren't caused by any structural abnormalities of the heart.

50/50

Approximately 50% of people over age 50 have innocent systolic murmurs. They're more common in women and in patients with hypertension. These systolic murmurs may not be so innocent when they occur in the presence of certain disease processes, such as anemia, fever, and thyrotoxicosis, because they can cause high-flow situations in which the accompanying systolic murmur isn't related to a cardiac defect.

The quality of innocent SEMs is variable. Other characteristics include soft intensity (less than a grade III/IV), short duration, distinctive start and end points, early diastolic timing and ending well before a normal S_2 split, and crescendo-decrescendo configuration. **(44)**

> Conditions such as pregnancy that require a high volume of blood circulating through the body may cause innocent systolic murmurs.

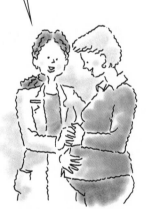

Pathologic systolic murmurs

Pathologic systolic murmurs are usually caused by:
- stenosis of the aortic valve or pulmonic valve
- insufficiency of the mitral valve or tricuspid valve
- interventricular septal defects.

Could be congenital

A patient may be born with a congenital defect or may acquire such a defect from such secondary conditions as rheumatic heart disease or idiopathic calcification of the valves. Because of the progressive nature of valve defects (for example, aortic stenosis), the timing and other characteristics of a systolic murmur can help to determine the severity of the disease.

Comprehensive considerations

When determining whether a systolic murmur is innocent or pathologic, it's important to consider the patient's history and symptoms and the results of various examinations and tests, including a chest X-ray, electrocardiogram (ECG), and echocardiography. Most innocent systolic murmurs occur in early systole or midsystole.

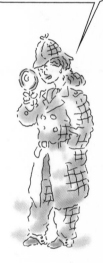

Consider the patient's history and symptoms and the results of various exams and tests when determining systolic murmur innocence.

Systolic murmur classifications

Systolic murmurs are classified as either *ejection* or *regurgitant*. SEMs are audible only during part of systole; that is, they start after S_1 and end before S_2 begins. (See *Auscultating for SEMs*, page 114, and *Tips for hearing SEMs*.) Because these murmurs are caused by aortic or

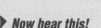

Now hear this!

Tips for hearing SEMs

A systolic ejection murmur (SEM) has a medium pitch that's heard best with the stethoscope's diaphragm. An SEM's intensity can be increased by maneuvers that increase blood volume or ejection velocity, such as having the patient raise his legs from a recumbent position, exercise briefly, or cough a few times.

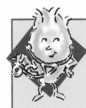

Location, location, location

Auscultating for SEMs

To determine whether a murmur intensifies, listen at the murmur's border. A systolic ejection murmur (SEM) is usually heard best along the left sternal border and, sometimes, over the aortic and mitral areas (shown below).

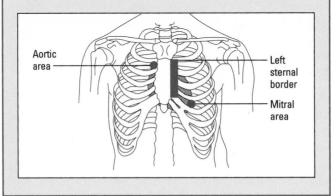

Aortic area

Left sternal border

Mitral area

Memory jogger

When characterizing systolic murmurs, use the mnemonic PISTOL:

Pitch

Intensity (grading)

Shape (configuration)

Timing (early systolic, midsystolic, late systolic, or holosystolic)

Other qualities (such as a description of the quality of the sound [for example, musical, cooing, blowing, or harsh])

Location

pulmonary abnormalities, they're divided into two categories: pulmonic SEMs and aortic SEMs. Regurgitant murmurs are audible throughout all of systole — that is, they start with S_1 and end with S_2.

Pulmonic systolic ejection murmurs

Pulmonic SEMs are caused by right ventricular outflow tract (RVOT) obstructions. RVOT obstructions are associated with pulmonic stenosis, narrowing of the artery or valve that may be *supravalvular, valvular,* or *subvalvular.* Regardless of location, the outflow obstruction causes turbulent blood flow that produces a midsystolic ejection murmur.

Early riser

The murmur begins early in systole — after S_1 and the opening of the diseased pulmonic valve. It ends before the S_2 closure component of the diseased pulmonic valve.

This murmur typically has a crescendo-decrescendo configuration that peaks in intensity in early systole, midsystole, or late systole, depending on the severity of the obstruction.

Supravalvular pulmonic stenosis murmurs

Supravalvular pulmonic stenosis, or *pulmonary artery branch stenosis*, is a type of RVOT obstruction that occurs above the pulmonic valve. (See *Understanding supravalvular pulmonic stenosis murmurs.*) The murmur is rarely accompanied by a pulmonic ejection sound (PES). **(45)** Supravalvular pulmonic stenosis is commonly associated with rubella syndrome or Williams syndrome (unusual facies, mental retardation, hypercalcemia).

Sound characteristics

Supravalvular pulmonic stenosis murmurs are usually heard over much of the thorax. (See *Auscultating for supravalvular pulmonic stenosis murmurs.*)

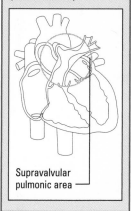

Understanding supravalvular pulmonic stenosis murmurs

Supravalvular pulmonic stenosis murmurs occur in the area slightly above the pulmonic artery (shown below).

Supravalvular pulmonic area

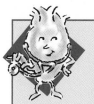

Location, location, location

Auscultating for supravalvular pulmonic stenosis murmurs

You can auscultate for supravalvular pulmonic stenosis murmurs over much of the thorax. This area is highlighted in the illustration below.

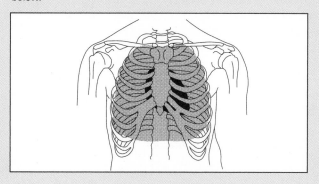

Supravalvular pulmonic stenosis murmurs on PCG and ECG

The supravalvular pulmonic stenosis murmur has a crescendo-decrescendo configuration. Note that the murmur begins just after the QRS complex and ends before the T wave begins, as shown on the photocardiogram (PCG) and electrocardiogram (ECG) representation below.

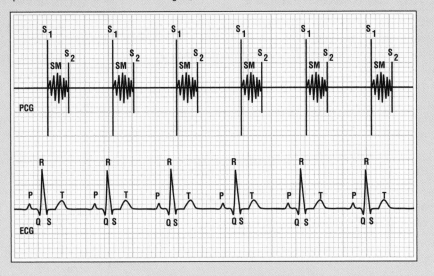

Other characteristics include:
- variable intensity and duration
- medium pitch that's heard best with the diaphragm of the stethoscope
- harsh quality
- systolic timing beginning after S_1 and ending before a normal S_2 split (see *Supravalvular pulmonic stenosis murmurs on PCG and ECG*)
- location on an ECG starting just after the QRS complex begins and ending just before the T wave ends
- crescendo-decrescendo configuration that's occasionally continuous. **(46)**

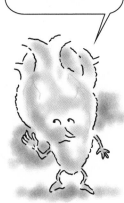

You can best hear RVOT obstruction murmurs with the diaphragm of the stethoscope.

Valvular pulmonic stenosis murmurs

A valvular pulmonic stenosis (or *pulmonic valve stenosis*) murmur is the most common type and accounts for more than 90% of pulmonic stenosis cases. It results from congenital pulmonic valvular stenosis and is commonly associated with other congenital heart defects. (See *Understanding valvular pulmonic stenosis murmurs*.) In mild pulmonic valve stenosis, S_1 is normal. The murmur begins after S_1 with a right-sided PES as the pulmonic valve abruptly stops opening. Remember, the PES is the only right-sided heart sound that increases in intensity during expiration and becomes less audible during inspiration. The murmur intensifies after the PES and peaks in midsystole; then it begins to fade. It ends before S_2. **(47)**

Raising the grade

In severe valvular pulmonic stenosis, the pressure gradient across the pulmonic valve increases. An increased pressure gradient causes the PES to be heard earlier; it may even fuse with S_1. Right ventricular ejection time is also prolonged. Consequently, the murmur has a longer crescendo and the intensity peaks later in systole. The prolonged right ventricular ejection time also causes a delay, creating a wide S_2 split. Usually, as the stenosis becomes more severe, the murmur's duration lengthens and its configuration becomes more asymmetrical.

Sound characteristics

Valvular pulmonic stenosis murmurs are heard best near the heart's base, over the pulmonic area. (See *Auscultating for valvular pulmonic stenosis murmurs*, page 118.)
    Other characteristics include:
• radiation toward the left neck or the left shoulder
• soft intensity that becomes louder with a palpable thrill toward the left neck and shoulder as stenosis becomes more severe
• short duration that increases as stenosis worsens
• medium pitch that's heard best with the diaphragm of the stethoscope
• harsh quality
• midsystolic timing ending before a normal S_2 split
• accompanied by a PES that diminishes or disappears with inspiration
• location on an ECG beginning after the QRS complex and ending before the end of the T wave
• crescendo-decrescendo configuration

Understanding valvular pulmonic stenosis murmurs

The pulmonic valvular area (shown below) produces a valvular pulmonic stenosis murmur.

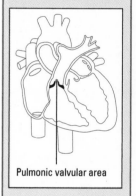

Pulmonic valvular area

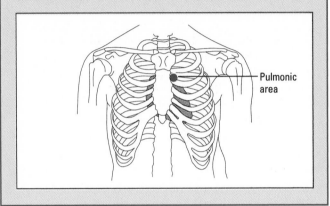

Location, location, location

Auscultating for valvular pulmonic stenosis murmurs

When auscultating for valvular pulmonic stenosis murmurs, place the stethoscope over the pulmonic area at the left sternal border (shown below).

Pulmonic area

• diamond-shaped (mild valvular pulmonic stenosis murmur
• kite-shaped (severe pulmonic valvular stenosis murmur). **(48)**

Subvalvular pulmonic stenosis murmurs

When an RVOT obstruction is subvalvular, or beneath the pulmonic valve, a midsystolic ejection murmur sounds the same as a pulmonic valvular stenosis murmur. (See *Understanding subvalvular pulmonic stenosis murmurs.*) However, this type of murmur isn't initiated by a PES. **(49)** Subvalvular pulmonic stenosis is uncommon and is associated with ventricular septal defects (VSDs) such as tetralogy of Fallot. When the subvalvular obstruction is associated with a VSD, the murmur is more complex.

My investigation reveals that the subvalvular pulmonic stenosis murmur is more complex in character, especially when associated with a VSD.

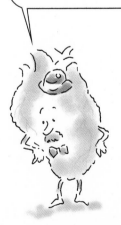

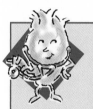

Location, location, location

Auscultating for subvalvular pulmonic stenosis murmurs

To listen for subvalvular pulmonic stenosis murmurs, place your stethoscope over the pulmonic area over Erb's point (shown below).

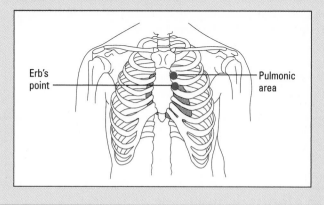

Erb's point — Pulmonic area

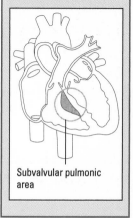
Sound characteristics

Subvalvular pulmonic stenosis murmurs are usually heard best over the pulmonic area and over Erb's point. They commonly radiate toward the left side of the neck, the left shoulder, or both. (See *Auscultating for subvalvular pulmonic stenosis murmurs.*)

Other characteristics include:
- soft intensity that becomes louder as stenosis worsens
- short duration that also increases as stenosis worsens
- medium pitch that's heard best with the diaphragm of the stethoscope
- harsh quality
- midsystolic timing starting after S_1 and ending before a normal S_2 split
- location on an ECG beginning after the QRS complex and ending before the end of the T wave **(50)**
- not initiated by a PES
- crescendo-decrescendo configuration.

Aortic systolic ejection murmurs

Aortic SEMs are caused by left ventricular outflow tract (LVOT) obstructions. LVOT obstructions are associated with aortic stenosis, which is a narrowing of the aorta through which the blood leaves the heart. Other causes of aortic SEMs include aortic dilation, aortic valve sclerosis, and increased aortic flow. Aortic stenosis may be *supravalvular*, *valvular*, or *subvalvular*. Regardless of location, the outflow obstruction causes turbulent blood flow that produces a midsystolic ejection murmur.

Subsequent to S₁

The murmur begins early in systole—after S_1 and the opening of the diseased aortic valve. It ends before the S_2 closure component of the diseased aortic valve. This murmur typically has a crescendo-decrescendo configuration that peaks in intensity in early systole, midsystole, or late systole, depending on the obstruction's severity.

Supravalvular aortic stenosis murmurs

Supravalvular aortic stenosis murmurs are usually congenital and are caused by aortic coarctation and fixed supravalvular stenosis. (See *Understanding supravalvular aortic stenosis murmurs*.)

A rare finding

Other causes of supravalvular aortic stenosis murmurs are rare but may include fibrous membranes and fibromuscular ridges above the aortic sinuses. These causes may produce a murmur similar to that heard with aortic valvular stenosis but louder, without an aortic ejection sound (AES), and heard best over the suprasternal area, aortic area, or right first intercostal space. **(51)**

Sound characteristics

Supravalvular aortic stenosis murmurs are usually heard best near the heart's base over the right first intercostal space, over the aortic area, and over the suprasternal notch. (See *Auscultating for supravalvular aortic stenosis murmurs*.)

Understanding supravalvular aortic stenosis murmurs

Supravalvular aortic stenosis murmurs affect the ascending aorta by creating either an hourglass-shaped internal constriction or a diffuse narrowing of the area.

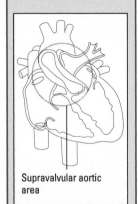

Supravalvular aortic area

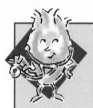

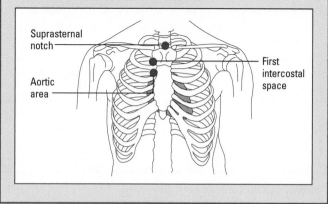

Location, location, location

Auscultating for supravalvular aortic stenosis murmurs

When auscultating for supravalvular aortic stenosis murmurs, place the stethoscope over the heart's base over the right first intercostal space, over the aortic area, and over the suprasternal notch. These areas are highlighted below.

Suprasternal notch

First intercostal space

Aortic area

Other characteristics include:
- radiation toward the right side of the neck, the right shoulder, or both
- typically grade III/VI to IV/VI intensity, decreasing in patients with left-sided heart failure
- increased duration as stenosis worsens
- medium pitch that's heard equally well with the diaphragm or bell of the stethoscope
- rough quality
- midsystolic timing that ends before the normal S_2 split
- not associated with AES
- location on an ECG beginning after the QRS complex and ending before the end of the T wave
- crescendo-decrescendo configuration (when an LVOT obstruction is above the aortic valve or supravalvular). **(52)**

Valvular aortic stenosis murmurs

Valvular aortic stenosis, most commonly known as *aortic valve stenosis*, can be congenital or can be acquired as a result of degenerative or rheumatic heart disease. (See *Understanding valvular aortic stenosis murmurs*.) If acquired from rheumatic heart disease, the mitral valve is usually also affected. Aortic stenosis produces an SEM that begins after S_1 and ends before S_2. **(53)**

Halting motion

After S_1, left ventricular pressure rises. The stenotic aortic valve halts its opening motion and produces a loud AES that's heard best near the heart's apex over the mitral area. The AES is followed by the murmur, which gradually intensifies until midsystole to late systole and then fades, ending before S_2.

Understanding valvular aortic stenosis murmurs

In valvular aortic stenosis, the aorta may have structural abnormalities, such as abnormal cusp formations, or calcification may occur.

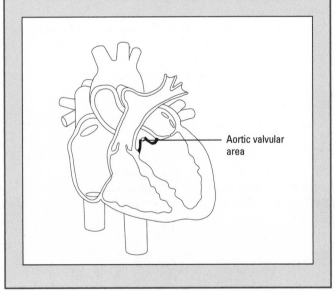

Aortic valvular area

Location, location, location

Auscultating for valvular aortic stenosis murmurs

When auscultating for valvular aortic stenosis murmurs, you can hear them best by placing the stethoscope over the aortic area, over Erb's point, or over the suprasternal notch. These areas are highlighted below.

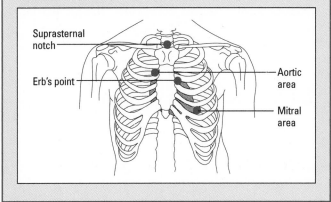

Sound characteristics

Valvular aortic stenosis murmurs are usually heard best near the heart's base over the aortic area, over Erb's point, near the heart's apex over the mitral area, or over the suprasternal notch. (See *Auscultating for valvular aortic stenosis murmurs*.) In older adults, these murmurs aren't as easy to find.

Other characteristics include:
• radiation toward the right side of the neck, the right shoulder, or both; possible palpable thrill over the aortic area and neck
• varying intensity from soft grade II/VI to rough grade IV/VI sound; typically grade III/VI to IV/VI intensity, decreasing in patients with left-sided heart failure
• increasing duration as stenosis worsens
• medium pitch that's heard equally well with the diaphragm or bell of the stethoscope
• rough quality that becomes harsher and louder with worsening stenosis

Valvular aortic stenosis may be congenital, or it may be acquired from degenerative or rheumatic heart disease.

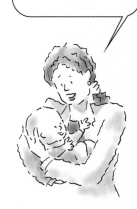

- midsystolic timing
- an AES heard shortly after S_1 (when present); AES following murmur, ending before a normal S_2 split
- severe stenosis (if an S_4 is heard before age 40)
- location on an ECG waveform beginning after the QRS complex and ending before the end of the T wave
- crescendo-decrescendo configuration. **(54)**

Subvalvular aortic stenosis murmurs

A subvalvular aortic outflow obstruction may be caused by fixed subaortic stenosis (which may present as a long, fixed segment or a short, fibrous ring) or hypertrophic cardiomyopathy, a genetic cardiac disorder. **(55)** This obstruction is produced by asymmetrical hypertrophy or thickening of the septum and abnormal anterior motion of the mitral valve leaflets during systole. (See *Understanding subvalvular aortic stenosis murmurs*.)

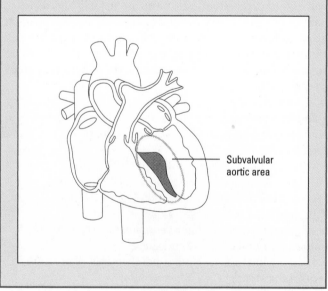

Understanding subvalvular aortic stenosis murmurs

Subvalvular aortic stenosis murmurs may be caused by a fibrous ring obstruction below the aortic valve or an abnormal hypertrophy of the septum.

Subvalvular aortic area

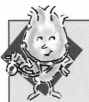

Location, location, location

Auscultating for subvalvular aortic stenosis murmurs

Subvalvular aortic stenosis murmurs are best heard over the heart's apex. Place your stethoscope over the tricuspid and mitral areas (shown below).

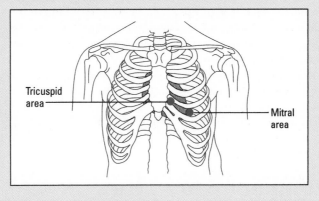

Tricuspid area

Mitral area

Sound characteristics

Subvalvular aortic stenosis murmurs are usually heard best near the heart's apex over the mitral and tricuspid areas. (See *Auscultating for subvalvular aortic stenosis murmurs*.)

Other characteristics include:
• usually no radiation toward the base, right side of the neck, or right shoulder
• typically grade III/VI to IV/VI intensity that increases as stenosis worsens
• variable duration
• medium pitch that's heard equally well with the bell or diaphragm of the stethoscope
• harsh or rough quality
• midsystolic timing peaking in midsystole and ending before a normal S_2 split or a paradoxical S_2 split
• location on an ECG beginning after the QRS complex and ending before the end of the T wave
• crescendo-decrescendo configuration. **(56)**

Differentiating subvalvular and valvular aortic stenosis murmurs

Because subvalvular and valvular aortic murmurs have similar characteristics, they may be difficult to differentiate. Here are some tips for distinguishing between them:
• A subvalvular hypertrophic cardiomyopathic murmur becomes louder during Valsalva's maneuver, whereas a valvular aortic stenosis murmur doesn't. Performing Valsalva's maneuver or having the patient stand up suddenly decreases venous return and left ventricular filling; this makes the left ventricle smaller, the obstruction more severe, and the subvalvular hypertrophic obstructive cardiomyopathic murmur louder.
• Having the patient squat increases peripheral vascular resistance and left ventricular filling; this maneuver decreases the pressure gradient across the aortic valve and decreases or obliterates the subvalvular hypertrophic obstructive cardiomyopathic murmur.

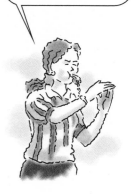

Tweet! Abnormal anterior motion of the mitral valve leaflets! That's 10 yards and a possible subvalvular aortic stenosis murmur!

Systolic insufficiency murmurs

There are three types of systolic insufficiency murmurs:
• tricuspid insufficiency murmurs
• mitral insufficiency murmurs
• VSD murmurs.

In reverse

An abnormality of either the tricuspid or mitral valve may result in backward turbulent blood flow during systole, so blood moves in a direction opposite that of the normal unidirectional flow pattern. Blood regurgitates through a defective, incompetent tricuspid or mitral valve into the left or right atrium, resulting in what's commonly called *tricuspid valve insufficiency* or *mitral valve insufficiency*, respectively.

Hole in one

An incompetent valve may be caused by a primary valvular disorder or may develop secondary to dysfunction of the valve's supporting structures, as in a VSD. A hole in the ventricular septum causes oxygenated and deoxygenated blood to mix and causes a VSD murmur.

Memory jogger

To remember the types of systolic regurgitation (insufficiency) murmurs (tricuspid, mitral, ventricular), use the mnemonic:

Some

Rich

Men

Take

Many

Vacations

Go configure

The regurgitant murmurs heard in patients with these valve disorders may be in early or late systole, or they may be holosystolic. Early systolic murmurs have a crescendo-decrescendo configuration, late systolic murmurs have either a crescendo or crescendo-decrescendo configuration, and holosystolic murmurs have a plateau shape.

Tricuspid insufficiency murmurs

Tricuspid insufficiency murmurs, also called *tricuspid regurgitation murmurs*, most commonly result from right ventricular dilation, which usually is caused by mitral valve disease or left-sided heart failure but may also be caused by pulmonary disease.

Occasionally, tricuspid insufficiency murmurs result from congenital valve malformations or from infective endocarditis, a right ventricular infarction, or trauma to the valve or its supporting structures. (See *Understanding tricuspid insufficiency murmurs*.)

Keep up the pace

A tricuspid insufficiency murmur can also be heard in a patient with a transvenous pacemaker because the pacemaker lead interferes with tricuspid valve closure, creating a tricuspid insufficiency-type murmur. The T_1 (tricuspid valve closure) intensity may be increased, normal, or decreased. **(57)**

Sound characteristics

Tricuspid insufficiency murmurs are usually heard best over the tricuspid area; in some patients, they're heard only during inspiration. (See *Auscultating for tricuspid insufficiency murmurs*, page 128.)

Other characteristics include:
• radiation to the right of the sternum
• soft intensity that increases during deep inspiration
• regardless of the tricuspid insufficiency murmur's etiology, increasing intensity during inspiration because venous return and right ventricular filling are increased, creating higher pressure gradients during systole
• long duration

Understanding tricuspid insufficiency murmurs

Tricuspid insufficiency murmurs are commonly caused by right ventricular dilation and an abnormal tricuspid valve, as shown below.

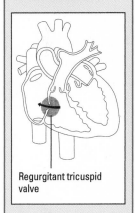

Regurgitant tricuspid valve

Location, location, location

Auscultating for tricuspid insufficiency murmurs

To auscultate for tricuspid insufficiency murmurs, place the stethoscope over the tricuspid area (shown below).

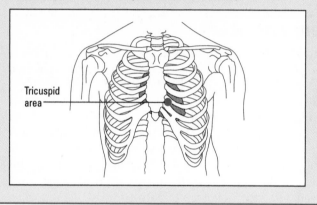

Tricuspid area

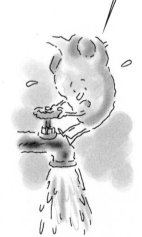

If only I could stop this flow! Blood regurgitating through a defective tricuspid or mitral valve results in insufficiency.

- medium pitch that's heard best with the diaphragm of the stethoscope (see *Tips for hearing tricuspid insufficiency murmurs*)
- scratchy or blowing quality
- rarely accompanied by a systolic thrill
- no correlation between its timing in systole or its intensity and the severity of the insufficiency
- systolic timing lasting from S_1 to S_2
- location on an ECG waveform beginning just after the QRS complex and ending after the T wave
- holosystolic
- plateau-shaped. **(58)**

Mitral insufficiency murmurs

Mitral insufficiency murmurs, also called *mitral regurgitation murmurs,* may be caused by congenital or acquired abnormalities of the mitral valve leaflets, the valve's supporting structures, or the left ventricle. An incompetent mitral valve causes backward blood flow during systole. The increased pressure at the aortic valve fa-

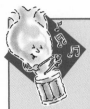

Now hear this!

Tips for hearing tricuspid insufficiency murmurs

Remember that tricuspid insufficiency murmurs are louder during inspiration. In some patients, this is the only time the murmur is audible.

How to hear the murmur

To enhance the murmur, have the patient breathe through his mouth slowly, quietly, and more deeply while sitting or standing. Caution the patient not to hold his breath because this negates the maneuver's effect. If a tricuspid insufficiency murmur is secondary to right-sided heart failure, right ventricular filling may be limited with inspiration; consequently, the murmur may not be intensified during deep breathing.

Understanding mitral insufficiency murmurs

Mitral insufficiency murmurs are caused by an abnormality of the mitral valve, as shown below, or left ventricle.

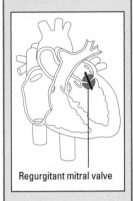

Regurgitant mitral valve

cilitates regurgitation of blood through the incompetent mitral valve into the low-pressure left atrium, producing a mitral insufficiency murmur. **(59)** (See *Understanding mitral insufficiency murmurs.*)

Sound characteristics

Mitral insufficiency murmurs are best heard over the mitral area. (See *Auscultating for mitral insufficiency murmurs*, page 130.)

Other characteristics include:
• appearance in early systole, midsystole, or late systole or holosystolic
• quality, duration, and radiation varying with extent, duration, and location of the disease process
• usually associated with mild to moderate insufficiency (if late).

Holosystolic mitral insufficiency murmurs

Holosystolic mitral insufficiency murmurs can be caused by the effects of rheumatic heart disease on the mitral

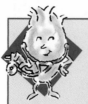

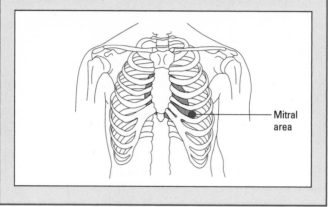

Location, location, location

Auscultating for mitral insufficiency murmurs

For all types of mitral insufficiency murmurs, including holosystolicmurmurs, acute mitral insufficiency murmurs, and mitral valve prolapse murmurs, place the stethoscope over the mitral area (shown below).

Mitral area

valve, by mitral valve prolapse, by left ventricular dilation, or by papillary muscle dysfunction.

Loud S₃

A loud S_3 usually accompanies moderate to severe mitral insufficiency; this sound is related not to ventricular failure but to the increased left ventricular volume in early diastole.

Sound characteristics

Holosystolic mitral insufficiency murmurs are usually heard best near the heart's apex over the mitral area. (See *Tips for hearing holosystolic mitral insufficiency murmurs.*)

Other characteristics include:
• radiation to the axillae or posteriorly over the lung bases
• variable intensity that usually isn't affected by respiration but may be somewhat diminished during inspiration

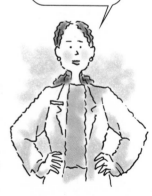

All mitral insufficiency murmurs are heard best over the mitral area.

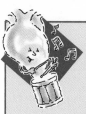

Now hear this!

Tips for hearing holosystolic mitral insufficiency murmurs

Holosystolic mitral insufficiency murmurs can usually be heard regardless of the patient's position, but grade I/VI to II/VI murmurs may be heard better with the patient in the partial left lateral recumbent position or after exercise.

- long duration
- medium to high pitch that's heard best with the diaphragm of the stethoscope
- accompanied by systolic apical thrill
- blowing quality
- systolic timing from S_1 to S_2
- location on an ECG just after the QRS complex to the end of the T wave
- holosystolic
- plateau-shaped. **(60)**

Acute mitral insufficiency murmurs

Acute mitral insufficiency murmurs are less common than chronic mitral insufficiency murmurs. Resulting from rupture of the chordae tendineae, papillary muscle, or both, these murmurs are occasionally caused by myocardial infarction but may also be caused by severe damage to the mitral valve from trauma or infection.

How it begins

An acute mitral insufficiency murmur is a decrescendo murmur that begins with mitral valve closure. **(61)** Its intensity decreases as ventricular and atrial pressures become equal during late systole. An S_4 is usually heard in acute mitral insufficiency.

Sound characteristics

Acute mitral insufficiency murmurs are usually heard best near the heart's apex over the mitral area. Other characteristics include:
• loud intensity (grade IV/VI to VI/VI if the murmur results from rupture of the chordae tendineae)
• accompanied by a systolic thrill
• medium to long duration
• high pitch that's heard best with the diaphragm of the stethoscope
• musical quality
• systolic timing
• location on an ECG beginning just after the QRS complex and ending just after the T wave
• commonly holosystolic and wedge-shaped (the wedge shape has a steeper decrescendo configuration). **(62)**

Mitral valve prolapse murmurs

Mitral valve prolapse is one of the most common valvular abnormalities found in adults. The murmur associated with mitral valve prolapse usually appears in late systole and is either isolated or accompanied by a nonejection midsystolic click (a click caused by the mitral valve prolapsing and ballooning up into the left atrium). Because of this, mitral valve prolapse murmurs are sometimes referred to as *click-murmur syndrome.* **(63)**

Sound characteristics

Mitral valve prolapse murmurs are usually heard best near the heart's apex over the mitral area. Other characteristics include:
• soft intensity (grade II/VI to III/VI)
• short duration
• high pitch that's heard best with the diaphragm of the stethoscope (see *Tips for hearing mitral valve prolapse murmurs*)
• musical quality (when loud, can be described as a whoop or a honk)
• late systolic timing (can be holosystolic)
• location on an ECG coinciding with the T wave and ending just after the T wave
• crescendo or crescendo-decrescendo configuration. **(64)**

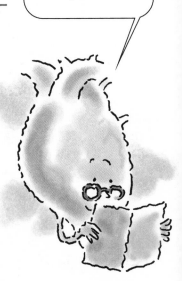

A mitral valve prolapse murmur is sometimes referred to as *click-murmur syndrome.*

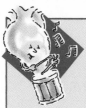

Now hear this!

Tips for hearing mitral valve prolapse murmurs

Here are some tips for improving your auscultation for mitral valve prolapse murmurs.

Positioning for timing
Ask the patient to stand, which decreases left ventricular volume. This allows a mitral valve prolapse murmur to be heard earlier in systole, to be louder, and to last longer. Having the patient squat increases left ventricular volume, which causes the murmur to be heard later in systole.

Disease-dependent direction
The direction in which the mitral valve prolapse murmur is transmitted across the chest wall depends on the disease process. For example, if the mitral valve's posterior leaflet is involved, blood flow might be directed more anteriorly and medially. Consequently, the murmur would be transmitted toward the heart's base and heard best over the aortic area and along the left sternal edge. If the anterior leaflet is incompetent, blood flow is directed posteriorly against the posterior left atrial wall, and the murmur is transmitted toward the left axilla and back.

Ventricular septal defect murmurs

A VSD is an opening, usually in the membranous portion of the ventricular septum, that allows direct communication between the ventricles. (See *Understanding VSD murmurs.*) Usually, VSDs are congenital, appearing at birth. Typically, blood shunts from left to right because of higher pressures in the left ventricle.

Sound characteristics

The VSD murmur is heard over the lower sternal border and, if loud, can be heard over the entire precordium. (See *Auscultating for VSD murmurs*, page 134.)

Understanding VSD murmurs
A ventricular septal defect (VSD) murmur occurs when a ventricular septum opening or defect allows blood to mix between the right and left ventricles, as shown below.

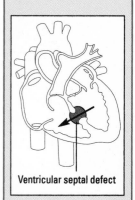

Ventricular septal defect

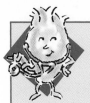

Location, location, location

Auscultating for VSD murmurs

For ventricular septal defect (VSD) murmurs, place the stethoscope over the lower left sternal border. If the murmur is loud, sometimes it can be heard over the entire precordium. These areas are illustrated below.

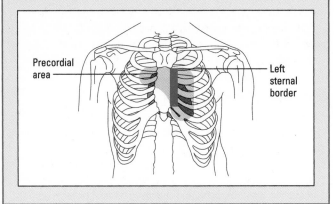

Precordial area — Left sternal border

Other characteristics include:
- palpable thrill along the lower left sternal border
- holosystolic
- widely split S_2 as the aortic valve closes early
- intensity and pitch that vary with the size of the VSD.

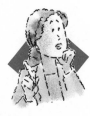

Quick quiz

1. Which of the following conditions causes a systolic insufficiency murmur?

    A.   Aortic valve stenosis
    B.   Pulmonic valve stenosis
    C.   Hypertrophic cardiomyopathy
    D.   Mitral insufficiency

Answer: D. Mitral insufficiency causes a systolic insufficiency murmur.

2. Which of the following conditions causes an SEM?
    A. Tricuspid insufficiency
    B. Mitral valve prolapse
    C. LVOT obstruction
    D. Ventricular septal defect

Answer: C. SEMs—but not systolic insufficiency murmurs—can be caused by LVOT obstructions, particularly those affecting the aortic valve.

3. Systolic murmurs aren't considered innocent in:
    A children.
    B. patients with thyrotoxicosis.
    C. thin-chested patients.
    D. pregnant women.

Answer: B. Systolic murmurs may not be innocent when they occur in the presence of certain disease processes, such as anemia, fever, and thyrotoxicosis.

4. An SEM is usually best heard:
    A. over the pulmonic area.
    B. over much of the thorax.
    C. along the left sternal border.
    D. at Erb's point.

Answer: C. An SEM is usually best heard along the left sternal border. It can also be heard sometimes over the aortic and mitral areas.

5. A midsystolic murmur can be heard in:
    A. mitral insufficiency.
    B. subvalvular aortic stenosis.
    C. tricuspid insufficiency.
    D. ventricular septal defect.

Answer: B. Subvalvular aortic stenosis is the only one of the above conditions with midsystolic timing. The rest may be late systolic or holosystolic.

6. The murmur associated with mitral valve prolapse usually appears in:
    A. early systole.
    B. late diastole.
    C. early diastole.
    D. late systole.

Answer: D. The murmur associated with mitral valve prolapse usually appears in late systole and is either isolated or accompanied by a nonejection MSC. Mitral valve prolapse is one of the most common valvular abnormalities found in adults.

Scoring

☆☆☆ If you answered all six questions correctly, magnificent! You're regurgitating the information about murmurs with ease.

☆☆ If you answered four or five questions correctly, bravo! You can obviously handle the pressure of systolic murmurs.

☆ If you answered fewer than four questions correctly, don't feel "ejected." There's time to go back and review this complex chapter.

Diastolic murmurs

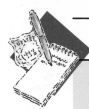

Just the facts

In this chapter, you'll learn:

♦ the way in which diastolic murmurs are produced

♦ differences between aortic and pulmonic insufficiency murmurs

♦ the characteristics of mitral stenosis murmurs

♦ the characteristics of tricuspid stenosis murmurs.

A closer look at diastolic murmurs

During auscultation, diastole is normally silent. You may, however, hear certain brief sounds that are also considered normal. These include the aortic component—pulmonic component (A_2-P_2) interval (as the aortic and pulmonic valves close) and a third heart sound (S_3) in a healthy person younger than age 20 (as the mitral and tricuspid valves open and the ventricles begin to fill).

Out of the ordinary

Occasionally, you may also hear a fourth heart sound (S_4) as the atria contract at the end of diastole to pump blood into the ventricles. S_4—considered an abnormal heart sound in all patients—is commonly heard in people with conditions that increase resistance to ventricular filling, such as a weak left ventricle.

A murmur heard during diastole is also considered abnormal. Unlike certain systolic murmurs, which can be innocent, diastolic murmurs almost always signal an underlying cardiac problem.

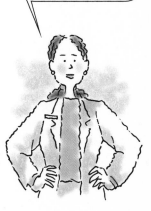

Unlike some systolic murmurs, diastolic murmurs are never innocent. If you hear a diastolic murmur, realize that the patient most likely has an underlying cardiac problem.

What time is it?

You can hear diastolic murmurs between the second heart sound (S_2) and the next first heart sound (S_1) — or, on an electrocardiogram (ECG) waveform, between the end of the T wave and the beginning of the QRS complex. When you hear a murmur, you first need to identify its timing. The timing is important information that can be used to help determine the murmur's cause.

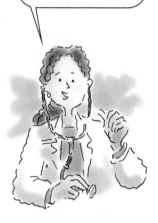

Listen carefully to determine exactly when during the cardiac cycle a murmur appears. The timing of the murmur provides an important clue about its cause.

Timing of diastolic murmurs

Diastolic murmurs are associated with ventricular relaxation and filling. They're described according to their timing during diastole. For example, a diastolic murmur may be described as *early diastolic, middiastolic, late diastolic,* or *holodiastolic* (occurring throughout diastole).

Early bird

An early diastolic murmur starts in S_2 and peaks within the early phase of diastole. Because the aortic and pulmonic valves close at the beginning of diastole, an early diastolic murmur usually results from insufficiency of the aortic or pulmonic valve.

Right in the middle

A middiastolic murmur occurs after S_2 and peaks in the middle phase of diastole. This is the time when the mitral and tricuspid valves open. Therefore, a middiastolic murmur usually signals stenosis of the mitral or tricuspid valve.

Fashionably late

A late diastolic murmur may also result from mitral or tricuspid stenosis. These murmurs begin and peak in the latter half of diastole, although they may extend to the next S_1. For this reason, a late-diastolic murmur may also be called a *presystolic murmur.*

The dominator

A holodiastolic, or pandiastolic, murmur starts with S_2 and extends throughout diastole. You'll typically hear this type of murmur in patients with patent ductus arteriosus or ventricular septal defects. (See *Don't believe everything you hear.*)

Ages and stages

Don't believe everything you hear

Because the third heart sound (S_3) and a holo-diastolic murmur are both low-frequency sounds heard after the second heart sound, you need to be careful not to confuse the two sounds during an auscultation assessment. Depending on the patient's stage of life, an S_3 may be normal.

S_3 results when decreased ventricular compliance accompanies increased ventricular volume during diastole. Because children and young adults normally have increased ventricular volume, an S_3 can be considered normal during these stages. Because of a high blood flow rate, a pregnant woman may also have an S_3. However, hearing a diastolic murmur during pregnancy is abnormal and warrants the doctor's attention.

In older adults, S_3 signals ventricular distress, an early sign of heart failure. You may frequently detect S_3 in patients with coronary artery disease, cardiomyopathy, and patent ductus arteriosus.

Conditions causing diastolic murmurs

Because the ventricles relax and fill during diastole, a diastolic murmur typically results from an insufficiency of the aortic or pulmonic valve or stenosis of the mitral or tricuspid valve.

Aortic insufficiency

Aortic insufficiency, also called *aortic regurgitation*, may cause either an early diastolic murmur or a middiastolic murmur.

Early diastolic murmur

Pressure in the aorta normally exceeds pressure in the left ventricle at the beginning of diastole. If the aortic valve fails to close properly, blood flows backward (retrogrades) across the incompetent aortic valve.

Counterproductive

This turbulent, backward flow produces an early diastolic murmur. In this instance, A_2 may sound normal or, if the patient has severe systemic hypertension, the sound may be accentuated. **(65)** (See *Understanding early diastolic aortic insufficiency murmurs.*)

Commonly associated with a systolic ejection murmur, this murmur may result from increased left ventricular stroke volume. Other possible causes include rheumatic heart disease, Marfan syndrome, osteogenesis imperfecta, or a dissecting aortic aneurysm. Leakage around a prosthetic aortic valve may also produce an early diastolic murmur.

Sound characteristics

You'll hear an early diastolic aortic insufficiency murmur best when auscultating near the base of the heart (over the aortic and pulmonic areas), over Erb's point, and near the apex of the heart (over the mitral area.) (See *Auscultating for early diastolic murmurs in aortic insufficiency.*)

Quiet, please!

This murmur usually has a soft intensity, so make sure to listen for it in a quiet environment. The murmur has a high pitch, which is heard best with the diaphragm of the stethoscope, and a blowing or musical quality. Beginning with A_2, the murmur may last through most of diastole. When looking at an ECG waveform, you'll see the murmur begin after the T wave and end just before the QRS complex. It has a decrescendo configuration. **(66)** (See *Tips for hearing early diastolic aortic insufficiency murmurs.*)

Middiastolic aortic (Austin Flint) murmur

If aortic insufficiency is severe, the backflow of blood from the aorta can interfere with the normal flow of blood across the mitral valve.

Causing a commotion

The blood flowing across the mitral valve becomes more turbulent, causing the mitral valve to vibrate. In turn, this produces a middiastolic and presystolic rumbling murmur, also known as an *Austin Flint murmur.* **(67)** (See *Understanding Austin Flint murmurs*, page 142.)

Understanding early diastolic aortic insufficiency murmurs

If the aortic valve fails to close properly, blood flows backward across the valve during diastole. This turbulent, backward flow across the incompetent valve produces the murmur.

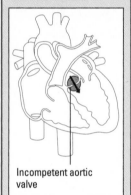

Incompetent aortic valve

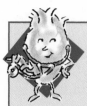

Location, location, location

Auscultating for early diastolic murmurs in aortic insufficiency

To hear an early diastolic murmur caused by aortic insufficiency, listen near the base of the heart over the aortic and pulmonic areas. You may also hear it by auscultating over Erb's point and the mitral area. These areas are highlighted on the illustration below.

If the murmur is associated with aortic root dilation or a dissecting aneurysm of the ascending aorta, the murmur may be louder along the right sternal border (between the second and fourth intercostal spaces) than along the left sternal border.

If you're listening for the murmur in an elderly patient or one who has chronic obstructive pulmonary disease, try listening near the apex of the heart for best results. If the murmur is loud, you may be able to hear it over most of the precordium.

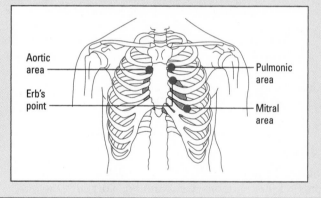

Aortic area

Erb's point

Pulmonic area

Mitral area

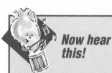

Now hear this!

Tips for hearing early diastolic aortic insufficiency murmurs

If you have difficulty hearing an early diastolic aortic insufficiency murmur, have the patient perform maneuvers to increase aortic diastolic pressure. These maneuvers include having the patient sit down, lean forward, and hold his breath after exhaling; having him squat; or giving him handgrip exercises to perform.

> If I have to have a murmur, at least it's one with a musical quality.

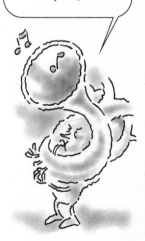

Sound characteristics

You'll hear an Austin Flint murmur best when auscultating near the apex of the heart, over the mitral area. (See *Auscultating for Austin Flint murmurs*, page 142.)

Ready to rumble

This rumbling murmur usually has a soft intensity and a low pitch, which is heard best with the bell of the stethoscope. When looking at an ECG waveform, you'll see this murmur just before the QRS complex. The presystolic portion of the murmur has a crescendo configuration,

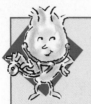

Location, location, location

Auscultating for Austin Flint murmurs

Because an Austin Flint murmur results from turbulent blood flow across the mitral valve, auscultate near the apex of the heart over the mitral area (shown below) to hear the murmur clearly.

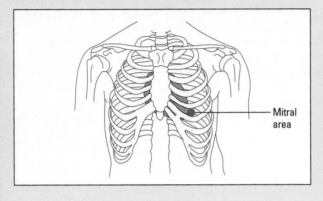

Mitral area

Understanding Austin Flint murmurs

In cases of severe aortic insufficiency, regurgitant blood from the aortic valve can meet, and interfere with, blood flowing into the ventricle across the mitral valve. The blood flowing over the mitral valve becomes more turbulent, most likely making the mitral valve vibrate, which produces an Austin Flint murmur.

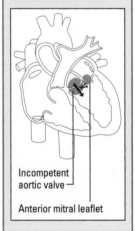

Incompetent aortic valve

Anterior mitral leaflet

while the middiastolic component has a crescendo-decrescendo configuration. **(68)**

Pulmonic insufficiency

During systole, the right ventricle ejects blood into the low-pressure pulmonary circulation. Normally, the pulmonic valve prevents the blood from returning to the right ventricle. In cases of pulmonic insufficiency, blood flows backward from the pulmonary artery into the right ventricle.

Too much of a good thing

A small amount of blood typically flows back across the valve in healthy adults, particularly in elderly people. However, an excessive backflow, or regurgitation, of blood can impair right ventricular function, leading to right-sided volume overload and heart failure.

Two types of pulmonic valve insufficiency murmurs may occur: Graham Steell's murmurs and normal pressure pulmonic valve murmurs.

Graham Steell's murmur

Because pressure in the pulmonary artery is normally quite low during diastole, significant regurgitation rarely occurs when the pulmonic valve is functioning normally. However, if a patient has pulmonary hypertension, the pulmonary artery dilates. This, in turn, dilates the pulmonic valve ring, resulting in a relative pulmonic insufficiency. (See *Understanding pulmonic insufficiency murmurs*.)

Feeling the pressure

The regurgitant flow of blood across the pulmonic valve produces a murmur that may be present throughout diastole. Called *Graham Steell's murmur*, it typically occurs only in cases of severe pulmonary hypertension, when systolic pulmonary artery pressure exceeds 60 mm Hg. **(69)**

Sound characteristics

The best place to hear a Graham Steell's murmur is along the left sternal border over the third and fourth intercostal spaces. The sound won't radiate to the right sternum. (See *Auscultating for pulmonic insufficiency murmurs*, page 144.)

Graham Steell's murmur has a loud intensity, which typically sounds louder during inspiration. It is characterized by its variable duration, high pitch (heard best with the diaphragm of the stethoscope), and blowing quality. Occurring in early diastole, this murmur begins with a loud P_2 and may include an ejection sound. It appears after the end of the T wave on an ECG and has a decrescendo configuration. **(70)**

> ### Understanding pulmonic insufficiency murmurs
>
> Pulmonic insufficiency murmurs, including both Graham Steell's murmurs and normal pressure pulmonic valve murmurs, result when high-velocity blood flows backward from a dilated pulmonary artery across an incompetent pulmonic valve.

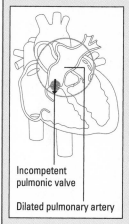

Incompetent pulmonic valve

Dilated pulmonary artery

You wouldn't be in this mess if your pulmonic valve would just do its job!

Hey, if you would keep your pressure down, my pulmonic valve would function just fine!

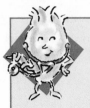

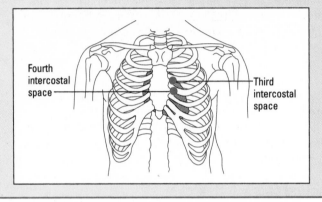

Location, location, location

Auscultating for pulmonic insufficiency murmurs

To hear either a Graham Steell's murmur or a normal pressure pulmonic valve murmur, listen along the left sternal border over the third and fourth intercostal spaces (shown below).

Fourth
intercostal
space

Third
intercostal
space

Normal pressure pulmonic valve murmurs

Murmurs may also result from idiopathic pulmonary artery dilation or from congenital pulmonary valve insufficiency. In either case, the pulmonary artery diastolic pressure remains normal.

Time to relax

Regurgitation occurs during isovolumic relaxation, after pressure in the right ventricle falls below pulmonary artery diastolic pressure. **(71)**

Sound characteristics

You'll hear a normal pressure pulmonic valve murmur best along the left sternal border over the third and fourth intercostal spaces. The sound won't radiate to the right sternum. (See *Tips for hearing pulmonic insufficiency murmurs*.)

Occurring in early diastole to middiastole, this type of murmur typically begins shortly after P_2. It has a rumbling quality with a soft intensity and brief duration. Unlike a

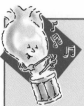

Now hear this!

Tips for hearing pulmonic insufficiency murmurs

Pulmonic insufficiency murmurs, particularly a normal pressure pulmonic valve murmur, intensify during inspiration. You'll hear the low-pressure regurgitant flow across the pulmonic valve as a brief crescendo-decrescendo, early diastolic murmur at the upper left sternal border. The sound becomes louder when the patient squats or takes a deep breath. The sound becomes softer when the patient exhales or performs Valsalva maneuvers. You may also note an S_3 or S_4 at the left mid-to-lower sternal border—a result of right ventricular hypertrophy or failure.

Graham Steell's murmur, it has a low pitch that's heard best with the bell of the stethoscope. When looking at an ECG, you'll see it begin after the T wave and end before the P wave. The murmur has a crescendo-decrescendo configuration. **(72)**

Mitral stenosis

Stenosis (narrowing) of the mitral valve usually results from chronic rheumatic heart disease caused by rheumatic fever. In rare instances, mitral stenosis may be congenital.

Narrow-minded and dysfunctional

Chronic inflammation of the mitral valve leads to scarring and calcification. Consequently, the valve assumes a funnel shape and stops functioning normally. Rapid, turbulent blood flow through the narrowed, rigid valve produces the murmur characteristic of this condition. (See *Understanding mitral stenosis murmurs.*)

Mitral stenosis is sometimes associated with mitral regurgitation, so you may also hear a systolic murmur. If mitral stenosis has caused pulmonary hypertension and right ventricular failure, tricuspid insufficiency may be the dominant murmur heard.

Understanding mitral stenosis murmurs

Mitral stenosis occurs when the mitral valve narrows or becomes obstructed. The narrowed valve reduces forward blood flow from the left atrium to the left ventricle, causing a murmur.

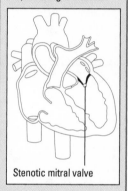

Stenotic mitral valve

Rheumatic fever can cause inflammation of the mitral valve that leads to scarring and calcification.

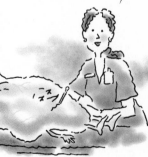

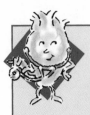

Location, location, location

Auscultating for mitral stenosis murmurs

To best hear a mitral stenosis murmur, auscultate over the mitral area (shown below) using the bell of the stethoscope.

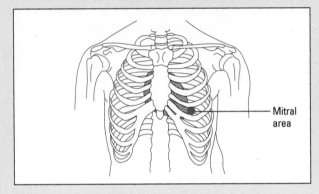

Mitral area

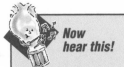

Now hear this!

Tips for hearing mitral stenosis murmurs

To enhance the sound of a mitral stenosis murmur, place the patient in a partial left lateral recumbent position. To further intensify the sound, have the patient perform maneuvers to increase cardiac output, such as raising his legs from a recumbent position, coughing several times, or performing some type of exercise for a few minutes.

Sound characteristics

The best location for hearing a mitral stenosis murmur is near the apex of the heart, over the mitral area. (See *Auscultating for mitral stenosis murmurs*.)

Stormy weather

With its variable intensity and duration, this murmur has a low pitch (heard best with the bell of the stethoscope) and a rumbling quality that sounds like thunder. (See *Tips for hearing mitral stenosis murmurs*.)

Snap to attention

Occurring shortly after S_2, the murmur begins with an opening snap. **(73)** An important diagnostic finding, the opening snap is a brief, loud sound that results when the stenotic valve suddenly halts its normal opening at the start of diastole. If the valve is calcified, S_1 is soft and the opening snap can't be heard. The murmur ends with a loud mitral component (M_1), or closing snap, which implies that the valve leaflets are mobile. The M_1 is usually palpable. **(74)**

The murmur has a crescendo-decrescendo configuration. You'll particularly notice the presystolic crescendo—the result of increased turbulence before systole—in patients having normal sinus rhythm. **(75)**

Sounds serious

The more severe the stenosis, the longer the duration of the murmur. In severe mitral stenosis, the murmur is holodiastolic; in moderate stenosis, it appears in early and late diastole. On an ECG waveform, the murmur begins just after the T wave and ends during the QRS complex.

Tricuspid stenosis

In tricuspid stenosis, the tricuspid valves become thickened and sclerotic, obstructing blood flow from the right atrium to the right ventricle.

Living large

This obstruction commonly causes the right heart to become enlarged which, in turn, may cause arrhythmias such as atrial fibrillation or flutter. Even if the patient has a normal sinus rhythm, you may notice signs of atrial enlargement, such as tall P waves on inferior leads. (See *Understanding tricuspid stenosis murmurs*, page 148.)

The social type

Tricuspid stenosis rarely occurs alone. Typically caused by rheumatic fever, it usually occurs along with a mitral valve defect and, occasionally, aortic valve disease. On rare occasions, tricuspid stenosis may result from a congenital defect of the tricuspid valve.

Sound characteristics

You'll hear the murmur resulting from tricuspid stenosis best when auscultating over the tricuspid area while the patient is in a partial left lateral recumbent position. (See *Auscultating for tricuspid stenosis murmurs*, page 148.)

Gone with the wind

The murmur has a soft intensity that increases during inspiration and fades or disappears during expiration. It has a variable duration, a low pitch (heard best with the bell of the stethoscope), and a rumbling quality.

> To differentiate a tricuspid stenosis murmur from a mitral stenosis murmur, remember that only the tricuspid stenosis murmur intensifies with inspiration.

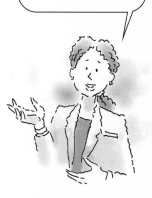

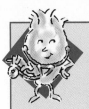

Location, location, location

Auscultating for tricuspid stenosis murmurs

Unlike a mitral stenosis murmur—which is heard best over the apex of the heart—you'll hear a tricuspid stenosis murmur best when you listen over the tricuspid area at the left sternal border (shown below).

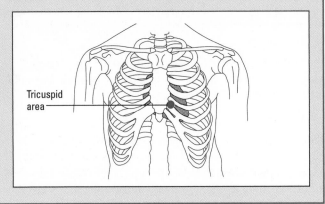

Tricuspid area

Understanding tricuspid stenosis murmurs

A tricuspid stenosis murmur results from a thickened and sclerotic tricuspid valve, usually the result of rheumatic fever.

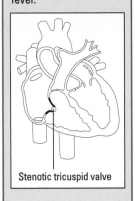

Stenotic tricuspid valve

The murmur appears in middiastole to late diastole, beginning shortly after a normal S_2 and ending just before S_1. An opening snap may precede the murmur, although it's seldom audible. However, unless the snap is obscured by a mitral stenosis murmur, it can usually be detected on a phonocardiogram. **(76)**

On an ECG waveform, the murmur begins just after the T wave and ends just before the QRS complex. In patients with normal sinus rhythm, the murmur has a late diastolic crescendo or crescendo-decrescendo configuration. **(77)**

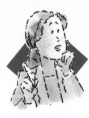

Quick quiz

1. Diastolic murmurs caused by aortic or pulmonic stenosis can usually be heard during:
   A. early diastole.
   B. middiastole.
   C. late diastole.
   D. holodiastole.

Answer: A. Because aortic and pulmonic valves close at the beginning of diastole, murmurs produced by dysfunctional aortic and pulmonic valves begin immediately after they close.

2. A diastolic murmur that starts after S_2 and extends throughout diastole is referred to as:
   A. early diastolic.
   B. middiastolic.
   C. late diastolic.
   D. holodiastolic.

Answer: D. Holodiastolic, or pandiastolic, murmurs start with an S_2 and extend throughout diastole. They commonly occur in patients with patent ductus arteriosus.

3. Murmurs caused by the regurgitation of blood from the aorta across the mitral valve are called:
   A. early diastolic aortic insufficiency murmurs.
   B. Austin Flint murmurs.
   C. Graham Steell's murmurs.
   D. mitral stenosis murmurs.

Answer: B. Austin Flint, or middiastolic aortic insufficiency, murmurs result when blood from the aorta regurgitates back into the ventricle before the ventricle contracts, causing the mitral valve to vibrate.

4. While auscultating a patient with severe pulmonary hypertension, you hear a murmur. This murmur is most likely:
   A. an Austin Flint murmur.
   B. a normal pressure pulmonic valve murmur.
   C. a Graham Steell's murmur.
   D. a mitral stenosis murmur.

Answer: C. Graham Steell's murmurs result when pulmonary hypertension causes the pulmonary artery to dilate. The high pressure then forces high-velocity regurgitant blood back across an incompetent pulmonic valve.

5. During auscultation, you hear a diastolic murmur that starts with an opening snap. An opening snap is diagnostic of:
   A. a tricuspid stenosis murmur.
   B. a mitral stenosis murmur.
   C. a normal pressure pulmonic valve murmur.
   D. a Graham Steell's murmur.

Answer: B. An opening snap is an important diagnostic feature of mitral stenosis. Although an opening snap may occur with tricuspid stenosis, it's rarely heard and is commonly obscured by a mitral stenosis murmur.

6. A patient with which type of diastolic murmur will most likely develop atrial flutter?
   A. Early diastolic aortic regurgitation murmur
   B. Pulmonic insufficiency (Graham Steell's) murmur
   C. Mitral stenosis murmur
   D. Tricuspid stenosis murmur

Answer: D. Tricuspid stenosis obstructs blood flow from the right atrium to the right ventricle. This commonly leads to an enlarged right atrium accompanied by atrial flutter or fibrillation. Therefore, a patient with a tricuspid stenosis murmur is most likely to develop atrial flutter.

Scoring

☆☆☆ If you answered all six questions correctly, excellent work! Everyone will be murmuring about your knowledge of diastolic murmurs.

☆☆ If you answered four or five questions correctly, good job! It sounds as if you have a firm grasp of these abnormal heart sounds.

☆ If you answered fewer than four questions correctly, don't despair. With a little more practice, you'll develop an ear for murmurs.

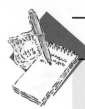

⓫

Continuous murmurs

Just the facts

In this chapter, you'll learn:
♦ the way in which continuous murmurs are produced
♦ conditions commonly associated with continuous murmurs
♦ methods for differentiating between a patent ductus arteriosus murmur and a cervical venous hum murmur
♦ the characteristics of a mammary souffle.

A closer look at continuous murmurs

Continuous murmurs begin in systole and persist without interruption throughout the cardiac cycle, late into diastole. These murmurs result from rapid blood flow through arteries or veins or from the shunting of blood. Shunting is caused by an abnormal communication between the high-pressure arterial system and the low-pressure venous system.

Causes for concern

Continuous murmurs may result from patent ductus arteriosus (PDA), mammary souffle, cervical venous hum, coarctation of the aorta or pulmonary artery, aorticopulmonary window, branch stenosis of the pulmonary artery, systemic or pulmonic arteriovenous (AV) fistulas, or atrial fistulas. Some of these produce a thrill, and many are associated with signs of right or left ventricular hypertrophy.

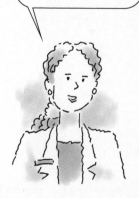

Continuous murmurs result from either the rapid flow of blood through arteries or veins or the shunting of blood from the arterial system to the venous system.

Conditions causing continuous murmurs

The three most common causes of continuous murmurs are cervical venous hum, PDA, and mammary souffle.

Cervical venous hum

Cervical venous hum murmurs—the most common continuous murmur—result when turbulent blood from the subclavian and internal jugular veins joins in the brachiocephalic vein before flowing downward into the superior vena cava. **(78)** (See *Understanding cervical venous hum murmurs.*)

Youthful expression

A normal, innocent occurrence in children, cervical venous hum murmurs rarely occur in adults. However, conditions causing hyperkinetic circulatory states, such as

---

Understanding cervical venous hum murmurs

The subclavian and internal jugular veins join to form the brachiocephalic veins, which feed into the superior vena cava. A cervical venous hum murmur occurs when rapid blood flow from the subclavian and internal jugular veins meets in the brachiocephalic veins.

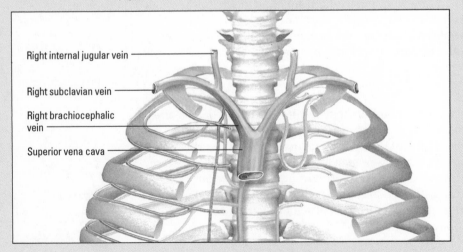

Right internal jugular vein

Right subclavian vein

Right brachiocephalic vein

Superior vena cava

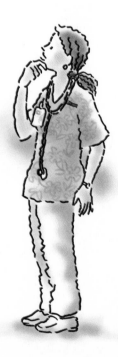

anemia, pregnancy, or thyrotoxicosis, may make the murmur more pronounced.

Sound characteristics

Although you may hear a cervical venous hum murmur on either side of the patient's neck, it's most audible on the right side. Have the patient sit with his head turned to the left while you auscultate the right side of his neck over the right supraclavicular fossa. Because the murmur has a low pitch, use the bell of the stethoscope while applying light pressure. (See *Auscultating for cervical venous hum murmurs.*)

Location, location, location

Auscultating for cervical venous hum murmurs

To best hear a venous hum murmur, have the patient sit with his head turned to the left. Applying very light pressure, use the bell of the stethoscope to auscultate over the right supraclavicular fossa, just above the clavicle. Ths area is highlighted in the illustration below.

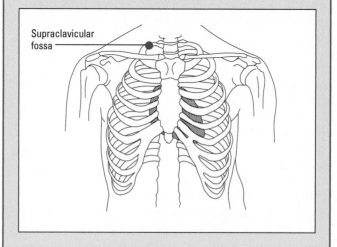

Supraclavicular fossa

Hum a few bars

Cervical venous hum murmurs have a soft quality and a faint intensity that increases during diastole, becoming louder between the second heart sound (S_2) and the first heart sound (S_1). **(79)** Lasting throughout the cardiac cycle, the timing is continuous (hence, the murmur's name). The murmur has a plateau shape in systole and a crescendo-decrescendo configuration in diastole.

Occasionally, the murmur may be loud enough to hear over the right sternal border, the sternum, or the left sternal border. In these instances, it can be mistaken for a murmur caused by PDA, aortic stenosis, or aortic insufficiency.

Disappearing act

When the patient performs Valsalva's maneuver, lies down, or turns his chin toward the stethoscope, the hum disappears. Applying pressure to the jugular vein on the side you're auscultating also obliterates the hum. Do this to differentiate between a venous hum and arterial or thyroid bruits, which don't disappear with pressure.

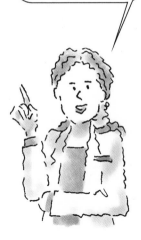

To test your finding of a cervical hum, apply pressure to the jugular vein during auscultation. If the sound disappears, it's a hum; if the sound persists, you're most likely hearing an arterial or thyroid bruit.

Patent ductus arteriosus

The ductus is a vascular channel between the aorta and the pulmonary artery. Open during fetal life, it normally closes shortly after birth. When the ductus remains open, as commonly occurs in premature infants, blood shunts from the high-pressure aorta to the low-pressure pulmonary artery. (See *Understanding PDA murmurs.*)

Reversal of fortune

Left untreated, a PDA may lead to irreversible pulmonary hypertension, which causes the shunt to reverse and flow from right to left. (This condition is known as *Eisenmenger's syndrome.*) A PDA usually presents as a systolic ejection murmur in newborns and develops into a continuous machinery murmur in older infants and children. **(80)**

Sound characteristics

PDA murmurs are best heard when auscultating over the first and second intercostal spaces to the left of the sternum. The sound to this area is limited when the intensity

Understanding PDA murmurs

When the ductus remains open after birth, blood shunts from the aorta, an area of high pressure, to the pulmonary artery, an area of lower pressure. A patent ductus arteriosus (PDA) murmur results.

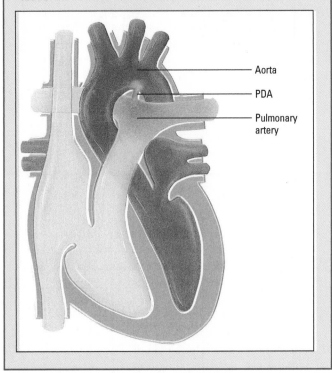

Aorta

PDA

Pulmonary artery

is faint. If the murmur is loud, you may hear the systolic component along the left sternal border and, perhaps, over the mitral area as well. A loud PDA murmur may radiate to the patient's back, between his scapulae. A thrill may also be palpable in loud PDA murmurs. (See *Auscultating for PDA murmurs*, page 156.)

Sizing things up

PDA murmurs have long durations, extending into diastole. The intensity is variable, roughly correlating with the ductus size. Typically, the murmur reaches maximum intensity late in systole and then fades during diastole. Exercise may increase the intensity and duration of a PDA murmur.

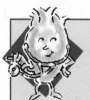

Location, location, location

Auscultating for PDA murmurs

Patent ductus arteriosus (PDA) murmurs can be heard when auscultating over the first and second intercostal spaces (shown below). Unlike venous hums, murmurs from PDA sound louder to the left of the sternum. If the patient has a loud murmur, you may hear the systolic component along the left sternal border and, occasionally, over the mitral area (also shown below).

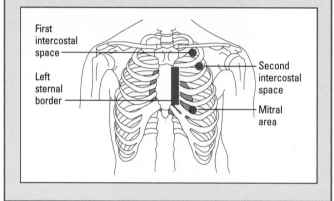

First intercostal space

Left sternal border

Second intercostal space

Mitral area

Pitch perfect

The pitch of PDA murmurs depends on the pressure gradient between the aorta and the pulmonary artery across the PDA. Small PDA murmurs and those in newborns usually have a high pitch, heard equally well with the bell or the diaphragm of the stethoscope, and a rough, machine-like quality. As the PDA gets larger, or in older infants and children, the pitch may be medium to low.

Drowning out the competition

The timing is continuous, beginning with, or shortly after, a normal S_1 and disappearing just before the next S_1. Because the murmur peaks in late systole, S_2 may be difficult to hear. If left ventricular ejection time is prolonged, S_2 may be paradoxically split. You may also hear a third heart sound (S_3) over the mitral area. **(81)** The murmur has a crescendo-decrescendo configuration. (See *Differentiating between continuous murmurs*.)

Differentiating between continuous murmurs

When trying to distinguish a cervical venous hum murmur from one caused by patent ductus arteriosus (PDA), remember that a venous hum is:

• loudest above the clavicle
• usually heard best to the right of the sternum
• obliterated if you press on the jugular vein or place the patient in a supine position
• truly continuous
• usually louder during diastole.

On the other hand, a PDA murmur is:
• heard best above the first and second intercostal spaces over the left sternal border
• loudest during late systole and fades during diastole.

Mammary souffle

Usually beginning in late pregnancy (second or third trimester) or during postpartum lactation, mammary souffle results from increased arterial blood flow to the breast. The sound typically disappears at the second postpartum month or at the end of lactation. The sound may also occur in young adolescent females because of increased blood flow to their developing breasts.

> I said, "I heard a souffle during my assessment," not "I want a soufflé for my breakfast."

Sound characteristics

The mammary souffle is a systolic or continuous sound that's heard best over the second intercostal space at the midclavicular line (over one or both breasts) or over the left sternal border. A continuous or diamond-shaped systolic murmur, the systolic component of the murmur begins after a slight delay following S_1. The murmur can be described as a soft blowing sound.

Take it lying down

Mammary souffle is best heard when the patient is lying down. If the patient sits upright or stands, or if you apply firm pressure to the diaphragm of the stethoscope, the sound disappears. The increased blood volume and enhanced cardiac output associated with normal pregnancy can also accentuate murmurs associated with stenotic heart valve lesions, such as mitral or aortic stenosis, if any are present.

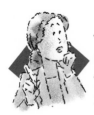

Quick quiz

1. The most common continuous murmur is a:
    A. cervical venous hum.
    B. PDA murmur.
    C. murmur from coarctation of the aorta.
    D. murmur from an AV fistula.

Answer: A. The most common continuous murmur is a cervical venous hum, which is innocent when it occurs in children.

2. When listening for a cervical venous hum, ask the patient to:
- A. perform Valsalva's maneuver.
- B. sit with his head turned to the left.
- C. lie down.
- D. sit with his head turned to the right.

Answer: B. Cervical venous murmurs become obliterated when the patient performs Valsalva's maneuver, lies down, or moves his head to the right.

3. To differentiate between a cervical venous murmur and an arterial or thyroid bruit:
- A. apply pressure to the jugular vein.
- B. listen with the diaphragm of the stethoscope.
- C. listen with the bell of the stethoscope.
- D. use very light pressure while listening with the stethoscope.

Answer: A. A cervical venous murmur disappears when you apply firm pressure to the jugular vein on the side where you hear the murmur; a bruit doesn't.

4. A mammary souffle murmur commonly occurs in:
- A. early pregnancy.
- B. children.
- C. late pregnancy.
- D. older women.

Answer: C. A mammary souffle murmur commonly occurs in late pregnancy and during lactation. It usually resolves by the second postpartum month or at the end of lactation. The murmur also may occur in young adolescent females because of increased blood flow to developing breast tissue.

Scoring

☆☆☆ If you answered all four questions correctly, incredible! You seem to have a continuous knowledge of murmurs that's most impressive.

☆☆ If you answered three questions correctly, well done! Everyone is humming about your success.

☆ If you answered fewer than three questions correctly, don't feel under pressure. Circulate back through the chapter and then try the quick quiz again.

12

Other auscultatory sounds

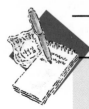

Just the facts

In this chapter, you'll learn:

♦ features of aortic and mitral prosthetic valves

♦ methods to detect a malfunctioning aortic or mitral prosthetic valve

♦ factors that cause a pericardial friction rub

♦ characteristics of a mediastinal crunch.

A look at other auscultatory sounds

In addition to the sounds already discussed, you may hear other sounds when performing a cardiac assessment. For example, if the patient has a prosthetic aortic or mitral valve, you'll hear sounds particular to the type of valve the patient has.

In this chapter, we'll look at the sounds produced by prosthetic aortic and mitral valves, a pericardial friction rub, and a mediastinal crunch. Becoming familiar with these sounds requires lots of practice. Be sure to take every opportunity to auscultate the hearts of patients who have prosthetic valves or those who have been diagnosed with valvular disease.

Understanding prosthetic valves

When a patient's heart valve malfunctions, usually because of stenosis or incompetence, he may receive a prosthetic valve. The most commonly replaced valves are the aortic and mitral valves. Tricuspid valves are occasionally replaced, but pulmonic valves rarely are.

Types of prosthetic valves

When a patient's heart valve malfunctions, he may undergo surgery to replace the malfunctioning valve with a prosthetic one. Here are the most commonly used valves.

Ball-in-cage valve

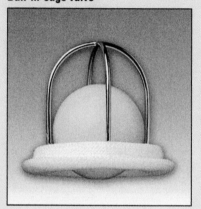

Starr-Edwards Silastic Ball Valve.
Photo courtesy of Edwards Lifesciences.

Tilting-disk valve

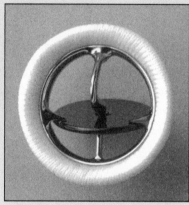

Medtronic Hall Mitral Valve.
Photo courtesy of Medtronic, Inc.

Bileaflet valves

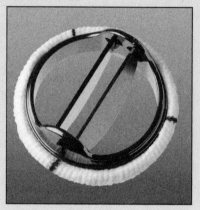

SJM Regent Valve.
Photo courtesy of St. Jude Medical.

The ball-in-cage valve uses a small ball, held in place by a metal cage, to keep blood flowing in a single direction. Although this valve is no longer inserted, you may still see a patient who has one. The most commonly used ball-in-cage valve was the Starr-Edwards valve.

The tilting-disk valve was developed as an alternative to the ball-in-cage valve. It has a hingeless design and contains open-ended, elliptical struts. This design feature reduces the risk of thrombus formation. The tilting-disk valve offers an improved forward flow of blood. It also causes minimal damage to blood cells. The most common tilting-disk valve includes Medtronic Hall valve.

The most commonly used valve, a bileaflet valve consists of two semicircular leaflets that pivot on hinges. The leaflets swing partially open and are designed to close so that an acceptale amount of regurgitant blood flow is permitted. In the United States, the St. Jude Medical valve is a commonly used bileaflet valve.

Types of prosthetic valves *(continued)*

Porcine valves

Bovine valves

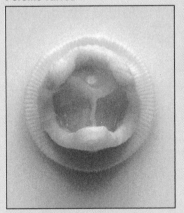

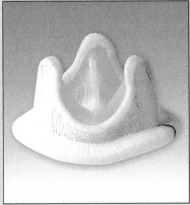

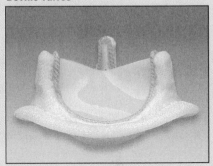

Carpentier-Edwards PERIMOUNT Pericardial
Bioprosthesis Valve.
Photo courtesy of Edwards Lifesciences.

Hancock II Aortic Bioprosthesis.
Photo courtesy of Medtronic, Inc.

Carpentier-Edwards Duraflex Low Pressure
Bioprosthesis Valve.
Photo courtesy of Edwards Lifesciences.

A porcine valve is made using a pig's aortic root that is sewn to a frame called a *stent*. The stent is commonly made from a plastic composite that is covered with a Dacron cloth. Porcine valves include the Medtronic Hancock II valve and the Carpentier-Edwards Duraflex Low Pressure Bioprosthesis valve.

Bovine valves are constructed using bovine pericardial tissue. These valves provide a complete opening for optimal hemodynamics.

Ionescu-Shiley constructed the first of these valves; however, that valve has been discontinued. The Carpentier-Edwards PERIMOUNT valve is now widely used.

Choices, choices

When undergoing valve-replacement surgery, a patient may receive a mechanical valve or a valve made from biological tissue (bioprosthetic valve). The main types of mechanical valves include:
- ball-in-cage valve
- tilting-disk (single leaflet) valve
- bileaflet valve. (See *Types of prosthetic valves*.)

Bioprosthetic valves may be made from animal tissue (heterograft or xenograft) or human tissue (homograft or allograft). Animal tissue valves are made from the pericardium of pigs (porcine valves) or cows (bovine valves). Human tissue valves are rarely used.

> More than 80 different models of prosthetic valves have been produced since the 1950s! But don't worry. You need to familiarize yourself with only the most common types.

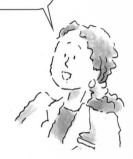

Pros and cons of mechanical and bioprosthetic valves

Doctors consider multiple factors when deciding which valve to place in a patient. The following chart lists the pros and cons of mechanical and bioprosthetic valves.

Valve type	Pros	Cons
Mechanical valves	• Offer high durability • Minimize the risk of calcification • Provide long function, possibly lasting throughout the patient's lifetime	• Pose an increased risk of blood clots, necessitating lifelong anticoagulation therapy • Carry an increased risk of infection • Damage blood cells • Provide poor hemodynamics • Place an increased demand on the heart, which decreases cardiac efficiency
Bioprosthetic valves	• Offer superior hemodynamics • Don't necessitate long-term anticoagulation therapy • Protect blood cells • Experience fewer structural problems • Offer a design closer to that of a natural valve • Conform to surrounding body tissues	• Provide good durability, but not as good as mechanical valves • Offer a shorter life span (10 to 15 years), necessitating replacement • Carry an increased risk of calcification (particularly in children and adults younger than age 40)

Young at heart

Mechanical valves are more durable and resist infection better than bioprosthetic valves. Because they last longer than bioprosthetic valves, a mechanical valve is usually the valve of choice for a younger patient. On the other hand, they're bulky and increase the risk of blood clotting. Therefore, patients with mechanical valves must take lifelong anticoagulant medication.

The issue with tissue

Bioprosthetic valves are a good alternative for some patients. These valves provide excellent hemodynamics, cause fewer problems than mechanical valves, and — because they're similar to human tissue — don't require lifelong anticoagulant medication. However, some of these valves are difficult to implant. They're also prone to calcification and, because they gradually deteriorate, they

Ages and stages

Choosing the right valve

Because mechanical valves last a long time—sometimes a patient's lifetime—they're usually inserted in children and adults younger than age 40. However, these valves shouldn't be inserted in women of childbearing age. That's because pregnant women are at risk for developing blood clots. Also, patients with mechanical valves must always take an oral anticoagulant medication, and warfarin (an anticoagulant) has been shown to cause birth defects when given during the first trimester of pregnancy.

Bio bias
Bioprosthetic valves are better suited for older patients. One reason is that calcification tends to occur on bioprosthetic valves, which can restrict blood flow or tear the valve leaflets. Patients younger than age 40 metabolize more calcium, placing them at a greater risk of developing calcification on a bioprosthetic valve. Furthermore, bioprosthetic valves gradually degenerate and must be replaced, making them less desirable for a patient who wants to avoid future surgery. However, because patients with bioprosthetic valves don't need anticoagulant medication, these valves may be a suitable option for women of childbearing age or those who are pregnant.

don't last as long as mechanical valves. (See *Pros and cons of mechanical and bioprosthetic valves* and *Choosing the right valve.*)

Identifying prosthetic valve sounds and murmurs

Prosthetic valves produce characteristic sounds and murmurs. Some of the sounds you'll hear depend on the type of valve being auscultated, while other sounds are universal, regardless of valve type. For example, all prostheses, regardless of type or position, produce closing clicks and some also produce opening clicks. (The ball-in-cage valves and small porcine valves produce the loudest sounds.) However, an aortic prosthetic valve doesn't change a normal first heart sound (S_1), and a mitral prosthetic valve doesn't change a normal second heart sound (S_2).

During auscultation, if you notice that a previously heard prosthetic valve sound has disappeared or become muffled, or if you hear a new murmur, suspect prosthetic valve malfunction.

Aortic prosthetic valves

The surgeon places a prosthetic valve in the aortic orifice so that it opens during systole and closes at the beginning of diastole. Each type of valve — ball-in-cage valves, tilting-disk valves, bileaflet valves, and porcine and bovine valves — produces distinctive sounds and murmurs. **(82)**

Hindering progress

Nearly all aortic prosthetic valves obstruct outflow to some degree, which causes a soft early systolic or midsystolic ejection murmur. Regardless of valve type, auscultate over the aortic, tricuspid, and mitral areas to hear these sounds best. (See *Auscultating for aortic prosthetic valve murmurs.*)

Aortic ball-in-cage valve

With a normally functioning aortic ball-in-cage valve, an aortic opening click follows and is louder than S_1. The sound is sharp and high-pitched, and it has a crisp quality. The intensity of the sound increases with rising cardiac output. An aortic closing click replaces the aortic component (A_2).

Sound characteristics

The murmur generated by an aortic ball-in-cage valve prosthesis typically has a loud intensity, making it easy to hear, and a medium pitch that's heard best with the diaphragm of the stethoscope. This midsystolic murmur has a variable duration and a crunchy, harsh quality.

Say no to outflow

Because ball-in-cage valves completely occlude outflow when closed, you won't hear a diastolic murmur. The interval between the aortic closing click and the pulmonic component (P_2) is similar to the normal A_2-P_2 interval, and it normally widens during inspiration. The murmur has a crescendo-decrescendo configuration.

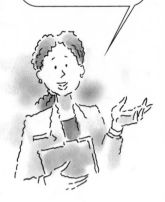

Not all change is good. If a patient with a prosthetic valve develops a new murmur or his heart sounds change, suspect valve malfunction.

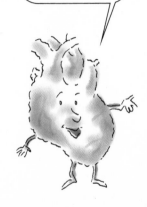

With my new ball-in-cage valve, I can really assert myself during an assessment.

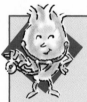

Location, location, location

Auscultating for aortic prosthetic valve murmurs

Aortic prosthetic valves typically produce systolic ejection murmurs that sound similar to mild aortic stenosis murmurs. You'll hear the sounds best when auscultating over the aortic area, the tricuspid area along the left sternal border, and near the apex of the heart over the mitral area. These areas are highlighted on the illustration below.

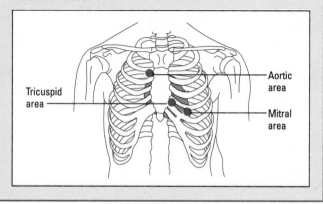

Detecting a malfunctioning aortic ball-in-cage valve

Common findings with a malfunctioning aortic ball-in-cage valve include a soft or absent aortic opening click as well as an absent closing click. You may also note a diastolic murmur and a prolonged systolic ejection murmur.

Aortic tilting-disk valve

With a normally functioning aortic tilting-disk valve, S_1 is unchanged. You may hear an aortic opening click as well as a closing click, although the closing click won't be as loud as the closing click heard with a ball-in-cage valve. The interval between the aortic closing click and P_2 should be normal.

Sound characteristics

The murmur generated by an aortic tilting-disk valve has a soft intensity (grade II/VI), a short duration, and a medium pitch that's heard best with the diaphragm of the stethoscope.

Sounds harsh

Appearing during systole, the murmur has a rough or harsh quality. The interval between the aortic closing click and P_2 is similar to the normal A_2-P_2 interval, although it widens during inspiration. The murmur has a crescendo-decrescendo configuration.

Detecting a malfunctioning aortic tilting-disk valve

If the patient has a malfunctioning aortic tilting-disk valve, you may discover some, or all, of these findings:
- an absent aortic closing click
- a diastolic murmur
- prolonged systolic ejection murmur.

Aortic bileaflet valve

A normally functioning aortic bileaflet valve produces a normal S_1. You should note a loud, distinct closing click; you may also hear an opening click.

Sound characteristics

The murmur generated by an aortic bileaflet valve has a soft intensity (grade II/VI), a short duration, and a medium pitch that's heard best with the diaphragm of the stethoscope. Appearing during systole, the murmur has a rough or harsh quality. The interval between the aortic closing click and P_2 is similar to the normal A_2-P_2 interval, and it widens during inspiration. The murmur has a crescendo-decrescendo configuration.

Detecting a malfunctioning aortic bileaflet valve

If an aortic bileaflet valve malfunctions, you may notice an absent aortic closing click, a diastolic murmur, or both. You may also hear a prolonged systolic ejection murmur.

Aortic porcine and bovine valves

When performing an auscultation assessment on a patient with an aortic porcine or bovine valve, you'll hear a normal S_2 with no opening click.

Sound characteristics

The murmur produced by an aortic porcine or a bovine valve has a soft intensity (grade II/VI), a short duration, and a medium pitch that's heard best with the diaphragm of the stethoscope. It also has a rough or harsh quality.

Closed-door policy

Because these valves completely occlude the outflow of blood when closed, you shouldn't hear a diastolic murmur. The interval between the aortic closing sound and P_2 is similar to the normal A_2-P_2 interval, and it widens during inspiration. The murmur has a crescendo-decrescendo configuration.

Detecting a malfunctioning aortic porcine or bovine valve

If an aortic porcine or bovine valve malfunctions, you may hear a diastolic murmur or a prolonged systolic ejection murmur.

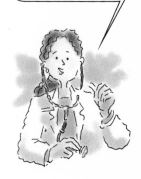

With normally functioning porcine and bovine valves, normal heart sounds rule. You should hear a normal S_2 with no opening click.

Mitral prosthetic valves

The surgeon places a prosthetic valve in the mitral orifice so that it closes at the beginning of systole and opens during diastole. Mitral prosthetic valves produce distinctive sounds and murmurs. **(83)** You'll hear the sounds best when auscultating over the mitral area, near the heart's apex, with the patient in a partial left lateral recumbent position. (See *Auscultating for mitral prosthetic valve murmurs*, page 168.)

Mitral ball-in-cage valve

Normally functioning mitral ball-in-cage valves produce opening and closing clicks.

Sound characteristics

During auscultation, you'll notice a loud, high-frequency opening click after a normal S_2.

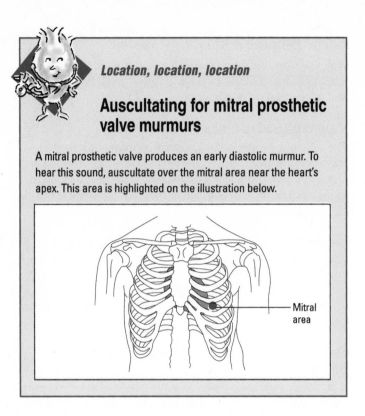

Location, location, location

Auscultating for mitral prosthetic valve murmurs

A mitral prosthetic valve produces an early diastolic murmur. To hear this sound, auscultate over the mitral area near the heart's apex. This area is highlighted on the illustration below.

Mitral area

Feeling jumpy

You may also hear several clicks of varying intensity, which result from the bouncing of the ball in the cage. The closing click is less prominent than the opening click.

Auscultation may reveal a short, soft (grade II/VI), rumbling diastolic murmur. Also, because the cage of this valve extends into the left ventricle and creates turbulent blood flow, you may hear a low-grade systolic murmur.

Detecting a malfunctioning mitral ball-in-cage valve

When a mitral ball-in-cage valve malfunctions in a patient with normal sinus rhythm, you may discover that the sounds normally associated with the valve vary in intensity. Other signs of valve malfunction include the appearance of a short interval between A_2 and the mitral opening click (indicating high left atrial pressure), a holosystolic murmur (indicating mitral regurgitation), and a change in the intensity and duration of the diastolic murmur (indicating mitral obstruction).

Mitral tilting-disk valve

A normally functioning mitral tilting-disk valve replaces the mitral component (M_1) with a mitral closing click.

Sound characteristics

The closing click produced by a mitral tilting-disk valve is distinct and high pitched. You may also hear a mitral opening click after a normal S_2. The patient may also have a short, soft, rumbling early diastolic murmur. The murmur sounds similar to a mitral stenosis murmur, except that it's brief and the presystolic component is absent.

Detecting a malfunctioning mitral tilting-disk valve

If a mitral tilting-disk valve malfunctions, you may notice that the mitral closing click has disappeared. Other possible findings include a new diastolic murmur, the intensification of a previously auscultated diastolic murmur, or a holosystolic mitral regurgitation murmur.

Mitral bileaflet valve

A mitral bileaflet valve produces a loud, high-pitched closing click that replaces M_1. Although rarely heard, a mitral opening click follows a normal S_2.

Sound characteristics

In addition to hearing a loud, high-pitched mitral closing click, you may also notice a short middiastolic rumble. Another possible finding is a short, soft, rumbling early diastolic murmur that sounds similar to a mitral stenosis murmur (except that this murmur is brief and doesn't have a presystolic component).

Detecting a malfunctioning mitral bileaflet valve

If a mitral bileaflet valve malfunctions, it may produce a holosystolic murmur, a new diastolic murmur, or both.

Mitral porcine and bovine valves

Because bioprosthetic valves are made from tissue, they generate sounds similar to those of a natural heart valve.

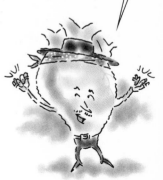

I've always enjoyed being unique. Now my tilting-disk valve has given me a closing click that's truly distinctive. Cha, cha, cha!

Sound characteristics

You won't hear an opening sound, and the closing sound is similar to a normal M_1. You may hear a short, soft, rumbling early diastolic murmur that sounds similar to a mitral stenosis murmur. However, this murmur is brief and the presystolic component is absent.

Detecting a malfunctioning mitral porcine or bovine valve

A malfunctioning mitral porcine or bovine valve may produce a holosystolic mitral regurgitation murmur, a diastolic rumble associated with mitral stenosis, or both. It may also cause an early to midsystolic murmur after S_2 that's followed by an opening sound.

Identifying other abnormal sounds

Other abnormal sounds you may identify during an auscultatory assessment include a pericardial friction rub and a mediastinal crunch.

Pericardial friction rub

When inflamed pericardial surfaces rub together, they produce a characteristic high-pitched friction noise known as *pericardial friction rub*. **(84)**

Rub a dub dub

A classic sign of inflammation of the pericardium (pericarditis), a pericardial friction rub may result from a viral or bacterial infection, radiation therapy to the chest, or cardiac trauma. Pericardial friction rubs commonly occur in patients who have had pericardiotomies. You may also hear one for a few hours, or a few days, following a myocardial infarction (MI). In addition to being audible, a pericardial friction rub may also be palpable in the tricuspid and xiphoid areas. (See *Auscultating for pericardial friction rubs.*)

Sound characteristics

A pericardial friction rub has a high pitch (heard best with the diaphragm of the stethoscope) and a grating or scratchy quality. Typically loud, it may grow even louder during in-

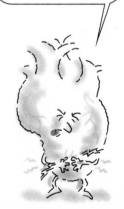

Ouch! This inflammation in my pericardium is really rubbing me the wrong way!

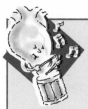

Now hear this!

Tips for hearing pericardial friction rubs

If you suspect that your patient has a pericardial friction rub, first have him lean forward to bring the heart closer to the chest wall. Alternatively, place him in a knee-chest position. Then, using the diaphragm of the stethoscope, auscultate initially over Erb's point. Listen intently as the patient exhales slowly and forcefully. Remain alert for high-pitched, leathery, scratchy sounds whenever the patient's heart contracts.

A friction rub may consist of between one and three components, which you'll hear during atrial systole, ventricular systole, or ventricular diastole. As a result, the sounds produced by the rub may coincide with the first or second heart sound..

Persist or cease?
To differentiate a pericardial friction rub from a pleural friction rub, have the patient hold his breath. The sound from a pericardial friction rub persists, while the sound from a pleural friction rub ceases.

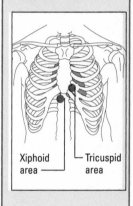

Location, location, location

Auscultating for pericardial friction rubs

To best hear a pericardial friction rub, auscultate over the tricuspid and xiphoid areas (shown below).

Xiphoid area — Tricuspid area

spiration. During each cardiac cycle, you may hear a pericardial friction rub during systole as well as during early and late diastole. **(85)** The diastolic component may last for only a few hours. (See *Tips for hearing pericardial friction rubs.*)

Mediastinal crunch

If air occurs in the mediastinum (such as in a pneumomediastinum), movements of the heart displace the air, producing a crunchy or crackling sound known as *mediastinal crunch*. Also called *Hamman's sign*, the sounds may occur randomly or in a consistent pattern. **(86)** Patients with mediastinal crunch commonly have subcutaneous emphysema (air trapped beneath the skin). As with stridor, treat mediastinal crunch as a medical emergency.

Location, location, location

Auscultating for mediastinal crunch

Remember that with mediastinal crunch, the sound is synchronized with the patient's heartbeat, not with his respirations. To auscultate this sound, place the patient in a left lateral decubitus position and then listen over the left sternal border (shown below).

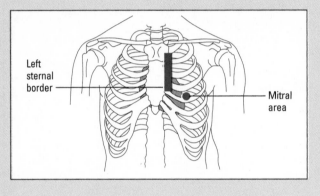

Left
sternal
border

Mitral
area

Sound characteristics

To hear the noises produced by mediastinal crunch, place the patient in a left lateral decubitus position and then auscultate along the left sternal border. (See *Auscultating for mediastinal crunch*.) You'll notice that the noises, which should have a crunching or scratching quality, are synchronous with the heartbeat. **(87)**

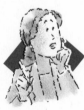

Quick quiz

1. The most advanced and most commonly used mechanical valve is the:

    A.   ball-in-cage.
    B.   tilting-disk.
    C.   bileaflet.
    D.   porcine.

Answer: C. Bileaflet valves are the most recent, and most commonly used, mechanical valves. The ball-in-cage valve is no longer inserted; the bileaflet valve was produced after the tilting-disk valve; and the porcine valve isn't mechanical.

2. If a 19-year-old patient requires a mitral valve replacement, he'll most likely receive which type of valve?
   A. Ball-in-cage
   B. Porcine
   C. Bovine
   D. St. Jude

Answer: D. Children and adults younger than age 40 have a high rate of calcium metabolism, which increases their risk of developing calcification on a bioprosthetic (bovine or porcine) valve. Ball-in-cage valves are no longer inserted. Therefore, the patient will most likely receive a St. Jude (bileaflet) valve.

3. A 25-year-old patient in her eighth week of pregnancy has mitral stenosis and needs a new valve. She will most likely receive a:
   A. tilting-disk valve.
   B. mitral porcine valve.
   C. homograft valve.
   D. St. Jude valve.

Answer: B. All mechanical valves, including the tilting disk and bileaflet (St. Jude) valves, require patients to take long-term anticoagulation therapy. This treatment is contraindicated in women who are pregnant or are of childbearing age because of the possibility of birth defects. Homograft valves are rarely used. Therefore, the patient will most likely receive a mitral porcine valve.

4. During an auscultatory assessment of a patient who suffered a myocardial infarction (MI) 2 days before, you hear a high-pitched, grating noise that grows louder during inspiration. You're hearing:
   A. pericardial friction rub.
   B. mitral stenosis.
   C. mediastinal crunch.
   D. crepitus.

Answer: A. Pericardial friction rubs are a classic sign of pericarditis; however, they may also occur following a pericardiotomy or an MI. Pericardial friction rubs produce high-pitched grating or scratching sounds that are best heard along the tricuspid and xiphoid areas. The sounds may increase during inspiration.

5.   During an auscultatory assessment, you hear scratchy or crackling sounds. To differentiate between a pericardial friction rub and a mediastinal crunch, you rely on the fact that:

    A.   pericardial friction rubs are synchronous with the heartbeat.

    B.   pericardial friction rubs are synchronous with respirations.

    C.   mediastinal crunches are synchronous with the heartbeat.

    D.   mediastinal crunches are synchronous with respirations.

Answer: C. Mediastinal crunches are synchronous with the heartbeat. Pericardial friction rubs — heard throughout the cardiac cycle — grow louder during inspiration and may disappear if the patient holds his breath.

Scoring

☆☆☆   If you answered all five questions correctly, outstanding! There's nothing insufficient about your knowledge of these other heart sounds.

☆☆   If you answered four questions correctly, super! You're really in tune with these valve sounds.

☆   If you answered fewer than four questions correctly, don't feel incompetent. A little more practice is all you need to master the ins and outs of valve sounds.

Cardiovascular disorders

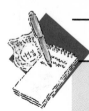

Just the facts

In this chapter, you'll learn:

♦ the pathophysiology of commonly encountered cardiovascular disorders

♦ common causes and assessment findings associated with the disorders

♦ heart sounds indicative of the disorders

♦ the best ways to hear these heart sounds on auscultation.

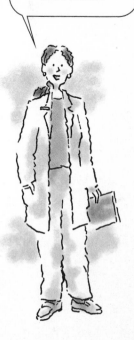

Cardiovascular disease remains the leading cause of death in the United States. Be sure to become familiar with common cardiovascular disorders as well as their distinctive heart sounds.

A look at cardiovascular disorders

Despite advances in disease detection and treatment, cardiovascular disease remains the leading cause of death in the United States. Heart attack, or myocardial infarction (MI), is the number one cause of cardiovascular-related deaths. If your patient is diagnosed with a cardiovascular disorder, you'll need to understand its disease process, what causes it, and what to look for. Each disease may produce distinctive heart sounds. The more you listen to patients' heart sounds, the more you'll feel comfortable and confident about understanding what you're hearing.

Abdominal aortic aneurysm

An abnormal dilation or ballooning in the arterial wall, abdominal aortic aneurysm most commonly occurs in the aorta between the renal arteries and iliac branches. More than 50% of all patients with untreated abdominal aneurysms die within 2 years of diagnosis, primarily from aneurysmal rupture. More than 85% die within 5 years.

What causes it

Aneurysms commonly result from atherosclerosis, which weakens the aortic wall and gradually distends the lumen. Other causes include:
• fungal infection (mycotic aneurysms) of the aortic arch and descending segments
• congenital disorders, such as coarctation of the aorta and Marfan syndrome (a multisystemic connective tissue disorder characterized by skeletal changes [such as abnormally long extremities], cardiovascular defects [commonly, dilation of the ascending aorta], and other deformities)
• trauma
• syphilis
• hypertension (in dissecting aneurysm).

Pathophysiology

Degenerative changes in the muscular layer of the aorta (tunica media) create a focal weakness, allowing the inner layer (tunica intima) and outer layer (tunica adventitia) to stretch outward. The resulting outward bulge is called an *aneurysm*. Blood pressure within the aorta progressively weakens the vessel walls and enlarges the aneurysm.

What to look for

Auscultation of the abdomen will reveal a "blowing" murmur over the aorta or a "whooshing" sound (bruit). Other symptoms may include:
• an asymptomatic pulsating mass in the periumbilical area
• abdominal tenderness on deep palpation
• lumbar pain that radiates to the flank and groin (a sign of imminent rupture).

Rupture indicators

If the aneurysm ruptures, look for:
• severe, persistent abdominal and back pain, mimicking renal or ureteral colic
• weakness
• sweating
• tachycardia
• hypotension.

Cardiac tamponade

In cardiac tamponade, a rapid rise in intrapericardial pressure equalizes right and left ventricular diastolic pressures, impairing diastolic filling of the heart. The rise in pressure usually results from blood or fluid accumulation in the pericardial sac.

Stretched to the limit

The fibrous wall of the pericardial sac can stretch to accommodate up to 2 L of fluid. If fluid accumulates slowly, such as in pericardial effusion caused by cancer, signs and symptoms may not be evident immediately. However, as little as 200 ml of fluid can create an emergency if it accumulates rapidly. Left untreated, cardiogenic shock and death can occur.

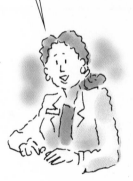

The pericardial sac can stretch to accommodate a large amount of fluid. If fluid accumulates slowly, signs and symptoms may not appear immediately.

What causes it

Cardiac tamponade may result from:
• effusion caused by cancer, bacterial infections, tuberculosis and, rarely, acute rheumatic fever
• hemorrhage caused by trauma, cardiac surgery, or perforation during cardiac or central venous catheterization
• hemorrhage from nontraumatic causes, such as rupture of the heart or great vessels or anticoagulant therapy in a patient with pericarditis
• pericarditis
• acute MI
• chronic renal failure during dialysis
• adverse reaction from procainamide, hydralazine, minoxidil, isoniazid, penicillin, or daunorubicin
• connective tissue disorders, such as rheumatoid arthritis, systemic lupus erythematosus, rheumatic fever, vasculitis, and scleroderma.

When cardiac tamponade has no known cause, it's called *Dressler's syndrome.*

Pathophysiology

In cardiac tamponade, the progressive accumulation of fluid in the pericardium compresses the heart's chambers. This obstructs blood flow into the ventricles and reduces the amount of blood that can be pumped out of the heart with each contraction.

Cramped for space

Every time the ventricles contract, more fluid accumulates in the pericardial sac. This further limits the amount of blood that can fill the chamber during the next cardiac cycle. Reduced cardiac output may be fatal without prompt treatment.

The amount of fluid necessary to cause cardiac tamponade varies greatly. It may be as small as 200 ml when the fluid accumulates rapidly or more than 2,000 ml if the fluid accumulates slowly and the pericardium stretches to adapt.

What to look for

Cardiac tamponade has three classic features, which are known as *Beck's triad:*

elevated central venous pressure with jugular vein distention

muffled heart sounds

pulsus paradoxus (inspiratory drop in systemic blood pressure greater than 10 mm Hg).

A late arrival

Unfortunately, Beck's triad is an extremely late finding. Pericardial friction rubs also aren't reliable indicators of tamponade; they're typically absent with large effusions.

Also look for

Other signs and symptoms include:
• orthopnea
• diaphoresis
• anxiety
• restlessness
• cyanosis
• weak, rapid peripheral pulse.

> **Memory jogger**
>
> To remember the three classic features, known as *Beck's triad,* that indicate cardiac tamponade, think **EMP-T.**
>
> **E**levated central venous pressure (with jugular vein distention)
>
> **M**uffled heart sounds
>
> **P**ulsus paradoxus
>
> =
>
> **T**riad

> Because Beck's triad is a late finding, you should keep your eye out for these earlier signs and symptoms.

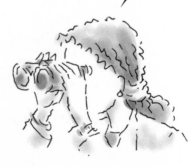

Cardiogenic shock

Sometimes called *pump failure*, cardiogenic shock is a condition of diminished cardiac output that severely impairs tissue perfusion. It reflects severe left-sided heart failure and occurs as a serious complication in some patients hospitalized with acute MI.

Cardiogenic shock typically affects patients whose area of infarction exceeds 40% of the heart's muscle mass. In such patients, the fatality rate may exceed 85%. Most patients with cardiogenic shock die within 24 hours of onset. The prognosis for those who survive is extremely poor.

What causes it

Most cases of cardiogenic shock result from acute myocardial ischemia. Other related causes include:
- toxicity to drugs such as doxorubicin
- infectious or inflammatory processes such as acute myocarditis
- certain drugs, such as beta-adrenergic blockers and calcium-channel blockers
- mechanical causes, such as valvular dysfunction, tamponade, or cardiomyopathy.

Patients with preexisting myocardial damage, arrhythmias, or diabetes are at increased risk for developing cardiogenic shock.

Pathophysiology

As cardiac output falls, aortic and carotid baroreceptors initiate sympathetic nervous system responses, which increase heart rate, left ventricular filling pressure, and peripheral resistance to flow, to enhance venous return to the heart.

A vicious cycle

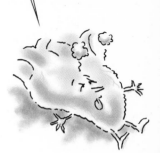

I've done my best to keep up my cardiac output by beating faster and working harder. But now I'm ready to collapse.

These compensatory responses initially stabilize the patient but later cause his condition to deteriorate as the oxygen demands of his already compromised heart rise. These events compose a vicious cycle of low cardiac output, sympathetic compensation, myocardial ischemia, and even lower cardiac output.

What to look for

The first step is to try to discover the cause of cardiogenic shock. For example, careful examination may reveal a mechanical cause, such as papillary rupture, valvular dysfunction, myocardial wall or septal rupture, cardiac tamponade, or aortic aneurysm. These conditions usually respond well to surgical intervention.

If you detect a loud murmur, suspect valvular dysfunction as the cause of the condition. Muffled heart tones along with jugular vein distention and pulsus paradoxus suggest tamponade.

Shocking signs

Cardiogenic shock produces signs of poor tissue perfusion, such as:
• cold, pale, clammy skin
• drop in systolic blood pressure to 30 mm Hg below the baseline, or a sustained reading below 80 mm Hg that isn't attributable to medication
• tachycardia
• rapid, shallow respirations
• oliguria (urine output less than 20 ml/hour)
• restlessness
• confusion
• narrowing pulse pressure
• cyanosis
• gallop rhythm and faint heart sounds.

Dilated cardiomyopathy

Dilated cardiomyopathy occurs when myocardial muscle fibers become extensively damaged. Disturbances in myocardial metabolism and gross dilation of the heart's chambers cause the heart to assume a globular shape. Dilated cardiomyopathy leads to intractable heart failure, arrhythmias, and emboli. Usually not diagnosed until its advanced stages, this disorder carries a poor prognosis.

What causes it

The primary cause of dilated cardiomyopathy is unknown. Although the relationship remains unclear, it occasionally occurs secondary to:
• viral or bacterial infections

- hypertension
- peripartum syndrome (related to toxemia)
- ischemic heart disease or valvular disease
- drug hypersensitivity or chemotherapy
- cardiotoxic effects of drugs or alcohol
- pregnancy (see *Taking a pregnant pause*)
- anemia
- thyrotoxicosis.

Pathophysiology

Dilated cardiomyopathy is characterized by both a grossly dilated, weak ventricle that contracts poorly as well as, to a lesser degree, myocardial hypertrophy. Increased volumes and pressures cause all four heart chambers to dilate. This leads to blood pooling, thrombus formation, and possible embolization.

Tired of leftovers

If hypertrophy coexists, the heart ejects blood less efficiently. A large volume of blood remains in the left ventricle after systole, leading to heart failure.

What to look for

The patient may develop:
- shortness of breath (orthopnea, exertional dyspnea, or paroxysmal nocturnal dyspnea)
- fatigue
- dry cough at night
- edema
- liver engorgement
- jugular vein distention
- peripheral cyanosis
- sinus tachycardia
- atrial fibrillation
- diffuse apical impulses
- pansystolic murmur (as a result of mitral and tricuspid insufficiency secondary to cardiomegaly and weak papillary muscles)
- third heart sound (S_3) and fourth heart sound (S_4) gallop rhythms.

> ### Taking a pregnant pause
>
> Dilated cardiomyopathy may develop during the last trimester of pregnancy or a few months after delivery. Its cause is unknown, but it occurs most commonly in multiparous women over age 30, particularly those with malnutrition or preeclampsia. In some patients, cardiomegaly and heart failure reverse with treatment, allowing a subsequent normal pregnancy. However, if cardiomegaly persists despite treatment, the prognosis is poor.

Endocarditis

Endocarditis (infection of the endocardium, heart valves, or cardiac prosthesis) results from bacterial or fungal invasion. Untreated endocarditis usually proves fatal but, with proper treatment, 70% of patients recover. Prognosis becomes much worse when endocarditis causes severe valvular damage, leading to insufficiency and heart failure, or when it involves a prosthetic valve.

What causes it

Causative organisms include group A nonhemolytic *streptococci*, *pneumococcus*, *Staphylococcus*, *Enterococcus* and, rarely, *gonococcus*.

Risky business

Most cases of endocarditis occur in patients who abuse I.V. drugs. Also at high risk are those who have prosthetic heart valves, a previous history of endocarditis (even in the absence of other heart disease), complex cyanotic congenital heart disease, or surgically constructed systemic pulmonary shunts or conduits. If endocarditis does occur in these patients, it's more likely to be severe and have a poor prognosis.

Patients with a moderate risk of severe infection include those who have an uncorrected patent ductus arteriosus, ventricular septal defect, primum atrial septal defect, coarctation of the aorta, or a bicuspid aortic valve. Patients who have valvular dysfunction from rheumatic heart disease or collagen vascular disease as well as those with hypertrophic cardiomyopathy also have a moderate risk of developing endocarditis.

Pathophysiology

Infection triggers the accumulation of fibrin and platelets on valve tissue.

A growing concern

Friable, wartlike, vegetative growths form on the heart valves, the endocardial lining of a heart chamber, or the endothelium of a blood vessel. These growths may cover valve surfaces, causing ulceration and necrosis, and may also extend to the chordae tendineae. Ultimately, the

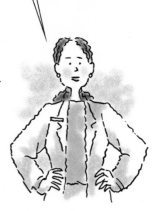

It's important to diagnose endocarditis early. When treated, 70% of patients recover. Without treatment, it's usually fatal.

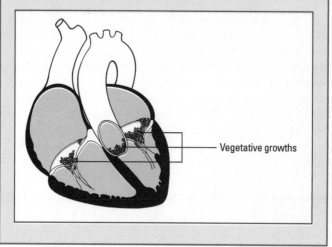

Effects of endocarditis

This illustration shows vegetative growths on the endocardium produced by fibrin and platelet deposits on infection sites.

Vegetative growths

growths may embolize to the spleen, kidneys, central nervous system, and lungs. (See *Effects of endocarditis.*)

What to look for

Early clinical features are usually nonspecific and include:
• weakness
• fatigue
• weight loss
• anorexia
• arthralgia
• night sweats
• intermittent fever (may recur for weeks)
• loud, regurgitant murmur (typical of underlying rheumatic or congenital heart disease)
• murmur that changes or appears suddenly, accompanied by fever.

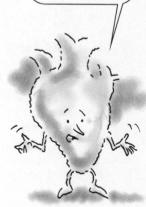

A fever, plus a new or changed heart murmur, is the classic sign of endocarditis.

Heart failure

When the myocardium can't pump effectively enough to meet the body's metabolic needs, heart failure results. Pump failure usually occurs in a damaged left ventricle but may also happen in a right ventricle. Usually, left-sided heart failure develops first. Heart failure is classified as:

Understanding left- and right-sided heart failure

These illustrations show how myocardial damage leads to heart failure.

Left-sided heart failure

Increased workload and end-diastolic volume enlarge the left ventricle (see illustration below). Because of lack of oxygen, the ventricle enlarges with stretched tissue rather than functional tissue. The patient may experience increased heart rate, pale and cool skin, tingling in the extremities, decreased cardiac output, and arrhythmias.

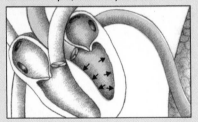

Diminished left ventricular function allows blood to pool in the ventricle and the atrium and eventually back up into the pulmonary veins and capillaries (as shown below). At this stage, the patient may experience dyspnea on exertion, confusion, dizziness, orthostatic hypotension, decreased peripheral pulses and pulse pressure, cyanosis, and an S_3 gallop.

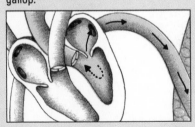

As the pulmonary circulation becomes engorged, rising capillary pressure pushes sodium (Na) and water (H_2O) into the interstitial space (as shown below), causing pulmonary edema. You'll note coughing, subclavian retractions, crackles, tachypnea, elevated pulmonary artery pressure, diminished pulmonary compliance, and increased partial pressure of carbon dioxide.

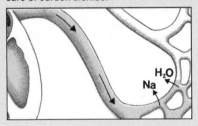

When the patient lies down, fluid in the extremities moves into the systemic circulation. Because the left ventricle can't handle the increased venous return, fluid pools in the pulmonary circulation, worsening pulmonary edema (see illustration below). You may note decreased breath sounds, dullness on percussion, crackles, and orthopnea.

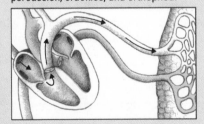

The right ventricle may now become stressed because it's pumping against greater pulmonary vascular resistance and left ventricular pressure (see illustration below). When this occurs, the patient's symptoms worsen.

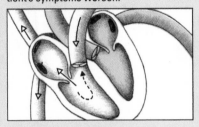

Right-sided heart failure

The stressed right ventricle enlarges with the formation of stretched tissue (see illustration below). Increasing conduction time and deviation of the heart from its normal axis can cause arrhythmias. If the patient doesn't already have left-sided heart failure, he may experience increased heart rate, cool skin, cyanosis, decreased cardiac output, palpitations, and dyspnea.

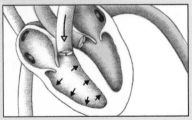

Understanding left- and right-sided heart failure *(continued)*

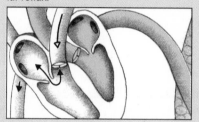 Blood pools in the right ventricle and right atrium. The backed-up blood causes pressure and congestion in the vena cava and systemic circulation (see illustration below). The patient will have elevated central venous pressure, jugular vein distention, and hepatojugular reflux.

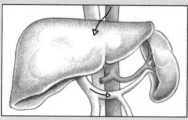 Backed-up blood also distends the visceral veins, especially the hepatic vein. As the liver and spleen become engorged (see illustration below), their function is impaired. The patient may develop anorexia, nausea, abdominal pain, palpable liver and spleen, weakness, and dyspnea secondary to abdominal distention.

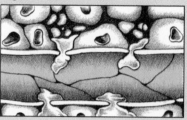 Rising capillary pressure forces excess fluid from the capillaries into the interstitial space (see illustration below). This causes tissue edema, especially in the lower extremities and abdomen. The patient may experience weight gain, pitting edema, and nocturia.

- acute or chronic
- left-sided or right-sided (see *Understanding left- and right-sided heart failure*)
- systolic or diastolic.

Performance evaluation

Symptoms of heart failure may severely restrict a patient's ability to perform activities of daily living. While advances in diagnosis and treatment have greatly improved the outcome for many patients, the prognosis still depends on the underlying cause and its response to treatment.

What causes it

Many cardiovascular disorders can lead to heart failure, including:
- atherosclerotic heart disease
- MI
- hypertension
- rheumatic heart disease
- congenital heart disease
- ischemic heart disease

- cardiomyopathy
- valvular diseases
- arrhythmias.

Disheartening causes

Noncardiovascular causes of heart failure include:
- pregnancy and childbirth
- increased environmental temperature or humidity
- severe physical or mental stress
- thyrotoxicosis
- acute blood loss
- pulmonary embolism
- severe infection
- chronic obstructive pulmonary disease.

Pathophysiology

The patient's underlying condition determines whether heart failure is acute or chronic. Typically, systolic or diastolic overload combined with myocardial weakness leads to heart failure.

Stressful situation

As stress on the heart muscle reaches a critical level, the heart's ability to contract declines and cardiac output falls. At the same time, venous blood flow to the heart remains the same, which causes the ventricles to fill with greater volumes of blood.

As cardiac output falls, the body responds by:
- increasing sympathetic activity
- releasing renin from the kidneys
- triggering anaerobic metabolism in affected cells
- inciting peripheral cells to extract more oxygen.

The long and short of the matter

The heart also tries to compensate. For example, as the end-diastolic fiber length increases, the ventricular muscle dilates and increases the force of contractions. Called the *Frank-Starling curve*, this is a short-term compensation measure. A long-term measure occurs as the ventricle hypertrophies. An enlarged ventricle allows the heart to contract more forcefully, ejecting more blood into circulation.

> Water is flowing in faster than I can bail it out. I think I'm beginning to fail!

What to look for

Clinical signs of left-sided heart failure include:
- dyspnea (initially upon exertion)
- paroxysmal nocturnal dyspnea
- Cheyne-Stokes respirations
- cough
- orthopnea
- tachycardia
- fatigue
- muscle weakness
- edema and weight gain
- irritability
- restlessness
- shortened attention span
- S_3 or S_4 heart sounds
- bibasilar crackles.
    The patient with right-sided heart failure may develop:
- edema (initially dependent)
- jugular vein distention
- hepatomegaly.

Hypertrophic cardiomyopathy

A primary disease of the cardiac muscle, hypertrophic cardiomyopathy is characterized by disproportionate, asymmetrical thickening of the interventricular septum, particularly the anterior-superior portion. It affects both diastolic and systolic function.

Obstructing traffic

The thickened septum obstructs blood flow through the aortic valve. As the papillary muscles become affected, mitral insufficiency occurs. The course of the disease varies; some patients progressively deteriorate, while others remain stable for several years. Sudden cardiac death can occur.

What causes it

Almost all patients inherit hypertrophic cardiomyopathy as a non-sex-linked autosomal dominant trait.

Pathophysiology

In hypertrophic cardiomyopathy, the left ventricular muscle enlarges, becoming stiff and noncompliant. Too little room remains in the ventricle to receive an adequate volume of blood during diastole, which reduces cardiac output. The heart compensates by increasing the rate and force of contractions. As left ventricular volume diminishes and filling pressure rises, pulmonary venous pressure also rises, leading to venous congestion and dyspnea.

What to look for

On auscultation, you may hear an S_3 or S_4 as well as a systolic ejection murmur. Heard best along the left sternal border at the apex of the heart, the murmur may have a medium pitch and is commonly intensified by Valsalva's maneuver.

Other clinical features include:
- angina pectoris
- arrhythmias
- dyspnea
- syncope
- heart failure
- pulsus biferiens
- irregular pulse (with atrial fibrillation).

Myocardial infarction

Characterized as an acute coronary syndrome, MI is an occlusion of a coronary artery that leads to oxygen deprivation, myocardial ischemia, and eventual necrosis. The extent of functional impairment and the patient's prognosis depend on the size and location of the infarct, the condition of the uninvolved myocardium, the potential for collateral circulation, and the effectiveness of compensatory mechanisms. In the United States, MI is the leading cause of death in adults.

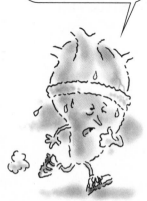

MI can result from any condition in which myocardial oxygen supply can't keep pace with the demand. Whew! I better slow down.

What causes it

MI can arise from any condition in which myocardial oxygen supply can't keep pace with demand, including:
- coronary artery disease
- coronary artery emboli
- thrombus
- coronary artery spasm
- severe hematologic and coagulation disorders
- myocardial contusion
- congenital coronary artery anomalies.

Hazardous conditions

Certain risk factors increase a patient's vulnerability to MI. These factors include a family history of MI; gender (men are more susceptible); hypertension; smoking; elevated serum triglyceride, cholesterol, and low-density lipoprotein levels; diabetes mellitus; obesity; sedentary lifestyle; aging; stress; and menopause.

Pathophysiology

MI results from prolonged ischemia to the myocardium with irreversible cell damage and muscle death. Functionally, MI causes:
- reduced contractility with abnormal wall motion
- altered left ventricular compliance
- reduced stroke volume
- reduced ejection fraction
- elevated left ventricular end-diastolic pressures.

What to look for

The patient experiences severe, persistent chest pain that's unrelieved by rest or nitroglycerin. He may describe the pain as crushing or squeezing. Usually substernal, pain may radiate to the left arm, jaw, neck, or shoulder blades. Other signs and symptoms include a feeling of impending doom, fatigue, nausea and vomiting, shortness of breath, cool extremities, perspiration, anxiety, hypotension or hypertension, palpable precordial pulse and, possibly, muffled heart sounds. (See *MI for the elderly guy [and gal!]*, page 190.)

Memory jogger

If you're assessing a patient and suspect he's experiencing a myocardial infarction but can't remember the classic signs, think of **CUSS**ing:

Chest pain (usually severe, persistent pain that's unrelieved by rest or nitroglycerin)

Upper body discomfort (usually substernal pain that radiates to the left arm, jaw, neck, or shoulder blades)

Shortness of breath

Several other possible symptoms (feeling of impending doom, fatigue, nausea and vomiting, cool extremities, perspiration, anxiety, blood pressure changes, palpable precordial pulse, and muffled heart sounds).

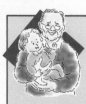

Pericarditis

Pericarditis is acute or chronic inflammation of the pericardium, the fibroserous sac that envelops, supports, and protects the heart. Acute pericarditis can be fibrinous or effusive, with purulent serous or hemorrhagic exudate. Chronic constrictive pericarditis characteristically leads to dense fibrous pericardial thickening.

Keeping company

Because pericarditis commonly coexists with other conditions, diagnosis of acute pericarditis depends on typical clinical features and the elimination of other possible causes. Prognosis depends on the underlying cause. Most patients recover from acute pericarditis, unless constriction occurs.

What causes it

Pericarditis may result from:
• bacterial, fungal, or viral infection (infectious pericarditis)
• neoplasms (primary or metastatic from lungs, breasts, or other organs)
• high-dose radiation to the chest
• uremia

- hypersensitivity or autoimmune diseases, such as rheumatic fever (the most common cause of pericarditis in children), systemic lupus erythematosus, and rheumatoid arthritis
- postcardiac injury, such as MI (which later causes an autoimmune reaction [Dressler's syndrome] in the pericardium), trauma, and surgery that leaves the pericardium intact but causes blood to leak into the pericardial cavity
- drugs, such as hydralazine and procainamide
- idiopathic factors (most common in acute pericarditis)
- aortic aneurysm with pericardial leakage and myxedema with cholesterol deposits in the pericardium (less commonly).

Pathophysiology

Inflammation causes the pericardium to become thickened and fibrotic. If it doesn't heal completely after an acute episode, it may slowly calcify, forming a firm scar around the heart. This scarring interferes with diastolic filling of the ventricles.

What to look for

Auscultation may reveal a pericardial friction rub. A classic sign, this grating sound occurs as the heart moves. To hear the friction rub best, firmly apply the diaphragm of the stethoscope to the left lower sternal border. Listen as the patient forcefully exhales while leaning forward or while he's on his hands and knees in bed.

Going through a phase

This rub occurs in three phases corresponding with atrial systole, ventricular systole, and ventricular diastole. However, it's uncommon for all three phases to be heard clinically. Occasionally, friction rub is heard only briefly or not at all.

Other signs and symptoms of pericarditis include:
- sharp, sudden pain that usually starts over the sternum and radiates to the neck, shoulders, back, and arms (unlike the pain of MI, pericardial pain is usually pleuritic, increasing with deep inspiration and decreasing when the patient sits up and leans forward)
- signs similar to those of chronic right-sided heart failure, such as fluid retention, ascites, and hepatomegaly (with chronic constrictive pericarditis).

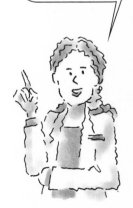

Unlike the pain of an MI, the pain of pericarditis increases with deep inspiration and decreases when the patient sits up and leans forward.

Restrictive cardiomyopathy

Characterized by restricted ventricular filling and failure to contract completely during systole, restrictive cardiomyopathy is a rare disorder of the myocardial musculature that results in low cardiac output and eventually endocardial fibrosis and thickening. If severe, it's irreversible.

What causes it

The cause of primary restrictive cardiomyopathy remains unknown. In amyloidosis, infiltration of amyloid into the intracellular spaces in the myocardium, endocardium, and subendocardium may lead to restrictive cardiomyopathy syndrome.

Pathophysiology

Left ventricular hypertrophy and endocardial fibrosis limit myocardial contraction and emptying during systole as well as ventricular relaxation and filling during diastole. As a result, cardiac output falls.

What to look for

Auscultation may reveal lung crackles, abnormal or distant heart sounds, and S_3 or S_4 gallop rhythms. Other findings include:
- fatigue
- dyspnea
- orthopnea
- chest pain
- generalized edema
- liver engorgement
- peripheral cyanosis
- pallor.

Rheumatic fever and rheumatic heart disease

A systemic inflammatory disease of childhood, acute rheumatic fever develops after infection of the upper respiratory tract with group A beta-hemolytic streptococci. Commonly recurrent, it mainly involves the heart, joints, central nervous system, skin, and subcutaneous tissues. If rheumatic fever isn't treated, scarring and deformity of cardiac structures result in rheumatic heart disease.

Worldwide, 15 to 20 million new cases of rheumatic fever are reported each year. The disease strikes most often during the cool, damp weather of winter and early spring. In the United States, it most commonly occurs in northern climates.

All in the family?

Because rheumatic fever tends to run in families, patients may be genetically predisposed to the disease. Environmental factors also seem to play a role. For example, in lower socioeconomic groups, the illness typically occurs in children between ages 5 and 15, probably because of malnutrition and crowded living conditions.

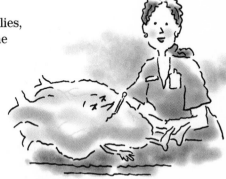

Untreated rheumatic fever can lead to rheumatic heart disease. I think you'd better rest.

Pathophysiology

Apparently, a hypersensitivity reaction to a group A beta-hemolytic streptococcal infection causes rheumatic fever. Because only about 3% of people infected with *Streptococcus* contract rheumatic fever, altered immune response probably influences its development or recurrence.

Getting complicated

Inflammation of the heart (carditis) develops in up to 50% of patients with rheumatic fever and may affect the endocardium, myocardium, or pericardium during the early acute phase. The extent of heart damage depends on where the infection strikes.

Myocarditis produces characteristic lesions called *Aschoff's bodies* in the interstitial tissue of the heart and also causes cells in the interstitial collagen to swell and fragment. This leads to the formation of progressively fibrotic nodules and interstitial scars.

A vegetative state

Endocarditis causes valve leaflets to swell and erode. Vegetative deposits also form on affected valves. Endocarditis typically strikes the mitral valve in females and the aortic valve in males. It may affect the tricuspid valve in either sex but rarely affects the pulmonic valve. Long-term effects include destruction of the mitral and aortic valves, which may lead to pericardial effusion and fatal heart failure. Of the patients who survive this complication, about 20% die within 10 years.

Pancarditis is the most serious and second most common complication of rheumatic fever. In advanced cases, patients may complain of dyspnea, mild to moderate chest discomfort, pleuritic chest pain, edema, cough, or orthopnea.

What to look for

In 95% of patients, rheumatic fever follows a streptococcal infection within a few days to 6 weeks and causes a temperature of at least 100.4° F (38° C). Most patients complain of migratory joint pain or polyarthritis. Swelling, redness, and signs of effusion—usually in the knees, ankles, elbows, and hips—also occur.

The most common sign of cardiac involvement is a new murmur (usually the result of valve insufficiency) and tachycardia out of proportion to fever. Other cardiac manifestations include heart failure and pericarditis.

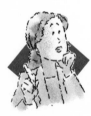

Quick quiz

1. During an auscultatory assessment of a cyanotic patient who's hemorrhaging, you hear muffled heart sounds. You suspect:
    A.   abdominal aortic aneurysm.
    B.   cardiac tamponade.
    C.   pericarditis.
    D.   rheumatic heart disease.

Answer: B. Muffled heart sounds are one of the three classic features, known as *Beck's triad*, of cardiac tamponade.

2. One-half of all cases of hypertrophic cardiomyopathy result from:
    A.   autoimmune disease.
    B.   malnutrition.
    C.   genetic predisposition.
    D.   infection.

Answer: C. One-half of all cases of hypertrophic cardiomyopathy result from genetic predisposition, whereas the rest result from an unknown cause.

3. A patient who had his mitral valve replaced 2 months previously has a temperature of 102.5° F (39.2° C). On auscultation, you hear a loud, regurgitant murmur. These findings suggest:
- A. endocarditis.
- B. pericarditis.
- C. dilated cardiomyopathy.
- D. restrictive cardiomyopathy.

Answer: A. Patients with prosthetic valves have a high risk of developing endocarditis. Typical findings include a loud, regurgitant murmur that may change or appear suddenly, usually accompanied by a fever.

4. Clinical signs of left-sided heart failure include:
- A. S_3 or S_4 heart sound.
- B. a friction rub.
- C. muffled heart sounds.
- D. a pansystolic murmur.

Answer: A. S_3 and S_4 heart sounds are among the clinical signs of heart failure.

5. When a patient is diagnosed with cardiomyopathy (either dilated, hypertrophic, or restrictive), you expect to hear:
- A. a pericardial friction rub.
- B. a loud, regurgitant murmur.
- C. a loud click.
- D. a gallop.

Answer: D. Cardiomyopathy causes ventricular gallops.

Scoring

☆☆☆ If you answered all five questions correctly, amazing! We wouldn't blame you if your heart were to swell with pride.

☆☆ If you answered four questions correctly, excellent work! You've surely put your heart into learning about these cardiac disorders.

☆ If you answered fewer than four questions correctly, don't be disheartened! Pump yourself up and go on to the next chapter.

Appendices and index

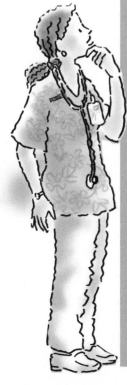

Common cardiac abbreviations

Here's a list of common cardiac abbreviations you may encounter when documenting heart sounds. Remember to use abbreviations cautiously and judiciously, as outlined by your facility's abbreviation policy.

A$_2$: aortic second sound

AAA: abdominal aortic aneurysm

ABG: arterial blood gas

ABP: arterial blood pressure

ACLS: Advance Cardiac Life Support

ACS: acute coronary syndrome

AFib: atrial fibrillation

AI: aortic insufficiency; aortic incompetence; apical impulse

AMI: acute myocardial infarction

A&P: anatomy & physiology

AP: apical pulse

AS: aortic stenosis

ASCVD: atherosclerotic cardiovascular disease

ASD: atrial septal defect

ASHD: atherosclerotic heart disease

AV, A-V: atrioventricular; arteriovenous

AVN: atrioventricular node

BBB: bundle-branch block

BCLS: basic cardiac life support

BP: blood pressure

CABG: coronary artery bypass graft

CAD: coronary artery disease

CBC: complete blood count

CCU: coronary care unit; cardiac care unit; critical care unit

CHD: coronary heart disease; congenital heart disease

CI: cardiac insufficiency; cardiac index

CK: creatine kinase

CO: cardiac output

CP: chest pain

CPR: cardiopulmonary resuscitation

CV: cardiovascular

CVA: cerebrovascular accident (stroke)

CVP: central venous pressure

CXR: chest X-ray

DBP: diastolic blood pressure

DM: diastolic murmur

DOE: dyspnea on exertion

Dx: diagnosis

ECG, EKG: electrocardiogram

ED: emergency department

EF: ejection fraction

EMD: electrical mechanical disassociation (cardiac arrest)

ER: emergency room

ESR: erythrocyte sedimentation rate

Hb, Hgb: hemoglobin

HCT: hematocrit

HDL: high-density lipoproteins

HEENT: head, ears, eyes, neck, throat

HR: heart rate

IABP: intra-aortic balloon pump

IAS: interatrial septum

ICD: implantable cardioverter-defibrillator

ICS: intercostal space

ICU: intensive care unit

INR: International Normalized Ratio (coagulation response time)

I&O: intake and output

IV: intravenous

IVC: inferior vena cava

JVD: jugular vein distention

JVP: jugular venous pulse

LA: left atrium

LAD: left anterior descending (coronary artery)

LBBB: left bundle-branch block

LCA: left coronary artery

LDL: low-density lipoproteins

LV: left ventricle

LVEDP: left ventricular end diastolic pressure

LVF: left ventricular failure

LVH: left ventricular hypertrophy

MAP: mean arterial pressure

MCL: midclavicular line

MI: myocardial infarction; mitral insufficiency

MSC: midsystolic click

MSL: midsternal line

MVP: mitral valve prolapse

MVR: mitral valve replacement

NSR: normal sinus rhythm

NYHA: New York Heart Association

O$_2$: oxygen

OS: opening snap

P$_2$: pulmonic second heart sound

PA: pulmonary artery

PAC: premature atrial contraction

Paco$_2$: partial pressure of arterial carbon dioxide

Pao$_2$: partial pressure of arterial oxygen

PAS: pulmonary artery systolic pressure

PAT: paroxysmal atrial tachycardia

PDA: patent ductus arteriosus

PE: physical examination; pulmonary embolism

PMI: point of maximal impulse

PTCA: percutaneous transvenous (or transluminal) coronary angioplasty

PVC: premature ventricular contraction

PVD: peripheral vascular disease

RA: right atrium

RBBB: right bundle-branch block

RBC: red blood cell

RCA: right coronary artery

RHD: rheumatic heart disease

RR: respiratory rate

RV: right ventricle

S$_1$: first heart sound

S$_2$: second heart sound

S$_3$: third heart sound

S$_4$: fourth heart sound

SA: sinoatrial (node)

Sao$_2$: arterial oxygen saturation

SB: sinus bradycardia

SBP: systolic blood pressure

SEM: systolic ejection murmur

SOB: shortness of breath

ST: sinus tachycardia

STAT: immediately

SV: stroke volume

SVI: stroke volume index

SVC: superior vena cava

SVT: supraventricular tachycardia

TI: tricuspid insufficiency

TIA: transient ischemic attack

TS: tricuspid stenosis

VF, vfib: ventricular fibrillation

VHD: valvular heart disease

VLDL: very-low-density lipoproteins

VS: vital signs

VSD: ventricular septal defect

VSS: vital signs stable

VT, V Tach: ventricular tachycardia

WBC: white blood cell

WNL: within normal limits

Auscultation findings for common disorders

Use this chart to review common cardiac disorders and their associated auscultation findings. Keep in mind that the patient may not present with every assessment finding listed for each disorder.

Disorder	Abnormal heart sounds
Abdominal aortic aneurysm	• Tachycardia • "Blowing" murmur over aorta or "whooshing" sound (bruit)
Aortic insufficiency	• Early diastolic murmur commonly with midsystolic murmur • "Cooing dove" or "musical" diastolic murmur signifies rupture or retroversion of an aortic cusp • Diminished A_2 • Early ejection click • Paradoxical S_2 split • S_3-S_4 gallop • Soft S_1
Aortic valvular stenosis	• Midsystolic murmur • Paradoxical S_2 split • Delayed A_2 and shortened A_2-P_2 interval • Aortic ejection sound radiates widely to neck and along great vessels • Systolic ejection sound if not severely stenotic
Atrial septal defect	• Wide, fixed S_2 split • Pulmonic ejection sound • Tricuspid component louder than mitral component
Cardiac tamponade	• Muffled or distant heart sounds • Pericardial friction rub (when associated with pericarditis)
Cardiogenic shock	• Gallop rhythm or faint heart sounds • Tachycardia
Dilated cardiomyopathy	• Irregular rhythm (with atrial fibrillation) • Pansystolic murmur • S_3 and S_4 gallop rhythms
Endocarditis	• Loud, regurgitant murmur • Murmur that changes or appears suddenly, accompanied by fever
Heart failure	• Tachycardia • Ventricular gallop (heard over the apex), S_3, or S_4

Disorder	Abnormal heart sounds
Hypertrophic obstructive cardiomyopathy	• Irregular rhythm (with atrial fibrillation) • S_3 and S_4 • Systolic ejection mumur that becomes louder with Valsalva's maneuver
Malfunctioning prosthetic aortic valve	• Long systolic ejection • Absent or softened aortic opening click • Absent or diminished aortic closing click • Diastolic murmur
Malfunctioning prosthetic mitral valve	• Holosystolic murmur • New diastolic murmur or change in intensity or duration of existing one • Diastolic rumble • Absent mitral closing click
Mitral insufficiency	• Holosystolic murmur • Decreased S_1 intensity • S_2 intensity increased • Accented P_2 • S_3 and S_4 gallop • Persistent A_2-P_2 splitting during expiration
Mitral stenosis	• Early and late diastolic murmur (with moderate stenosis) • Holodiastolic murmur (in severe stenosis) • Loud M_1 • Intensified S_1 except with a calcified valve, which produces a soft S_1 • Split S_2 • Opening snap except with a calcified valve • S_3 gallop
Mitral valve prolapse	• Late systolic or holosystolic murmur • Nonejection midsystolic click that's variable in intensity and timing • Precordial knock
Myocardial infarction	• S_3 and S_4 • S_1 and S_2 faint and poor quality • Paradoxical splitting S_2 with left ventricular dysfunction or left bundle-branch block (BBB) • Physiologic splitting S_2 with right BBB, ventricular septal defect, severe mitral insufficiency • Harsh holosystolic murmur, crescendo-decrescendo with palpable thrill if ventricular septal rupture

Disorder	Abnormal heart sounds
Patent ductus arteriosus	• Continuous murmur reaching maximum intensity during late systole • Murmur envelops S_2 • Paradoxical S_2 split • Diastolic flow rumble • S_3
Pericarditis	• Pericardial friction rub, which has both a systolic (loudest) and diastolic component • Scratchy, grating, superficial quality
Prosthetic aortic valve	• Systolic murmur • Aortic opening click • Aortic closing click • Interval between aortic closing click and P_2 that widens during inspiration
Prosthetic mitral valve	• Systolic murmur • Mitral closing click • Mitral opening click depending on valve type • Diastolic murmur depending on valve type
Pulmonary edema	• S_3 or S_4
Pulmonic insufficiency	• Early diastolic murmur intensified during inspiration • Loud P_2
Pulmonic valve stenosis	• Midsystolic murmur • Systolic ejection click • P_2 absent or diminished and delayed • Normal or widened S_2 split • S_4
Restrictive cardiomyopathy	• Abnormal or distant heart sounds • S_3 or S_4 gallop • Systolic murmur
Rheumatic heart disease, rheumatic fever	• Carditis or valvulitis • Carditis is detected by: – New murmur (usually mitral insufficiency) – Tachycardia out of proportion to fever – S_3 gallop • Valvulitis is detected by: – New or changing murmurs – Cardiac manifestations of heart failure and pericarditis (such as tachycardia, ventricular gallop, and pericardial friction rub)

Disorder	Abnormal heart sounds
Supravalvular aortic stenosis	• Midsystolic murmur • Normal S_2 split • No aortic ejection sound
Tricuspid stenosis	• Middiastolic to late-diastolic murmur, which increases during inspiration and fades during expiration • Normal S_2 or may be split during inspiration • Opening snap seldom heard
Ventricular septal defect	• Loud holosystolic murmur • Persistent A_2-P_2 splitting during expiration • Abnormal S_3 followed by short low-frequency diastolic murmur • Pulmonic ejection sound • Loud P_2

Glossary

A_2: aortic component of S_2

acute pulmonary hypertension: sudden increased pressure within the pulmonary circulation (above 30 mm Hg systolic and 12 mm Hg diastolic)

afterload: resistance that the left ventricle must work against to pump blood through the aorta

amplitude: magnitude or intensity of a sound or pulsation

aneurysm: sac formed by the dilation of a wall of an artery, a vein, or the heart

aortic ejection sound: opening sound of a stenotic aortic valve; it follows S_1 early in ventricular systole and appears just after the QRS complex on the electrocardiogram

aortic insufficiency: abnormal condition of turbulent backward blood flow through the aortic valve into the left ventricle during diastole

aortic stenosis: narrowing or constriction of the aortic valve or of the aorta itself

aortic valve: membranous folds that prevent blood reflux from the aorta into the left ventricle

aortic valvular stenosis: constriction of or damage to the aortic valve that restricts forward blood flow from the left ventricle to the aorta during systole

arteriovenous shunt: direct passage of blood from arteries to veins, bypassing the capillary bed; this can refer to a physiologic response of the body or to an abnormal condition sometimes caused by trauma or surgery

ascending aortic aneurysm: dilation of the thoracic portion of the aorta

asystole: absence of contraction of the heart

atelectasis: incomplete expansion of the lung tissue, usually caused by pressure from exudate, fluid, tumor, or an obstructed airway; may involve a lung segment or an entire lobe

atrial septal defect: imperfection, failure to develop fully, or absence of the dividing wall (septum) between the heart's atria

atrioventricular node: small mass of specialized cardiac tissue, located in the lower portion of the right atrium near the septum, that transmits electrical impulses from the sinoatrial node to the bundle of His

atrioventricular valves: valves between the atria and the ventricles, specifically, the tricuspid valve of the heart's right side and the mitral valve of the heart's left side

auscultation: act of listening to sounds made within the body; usually performed with a stethoscope

Austin Flint murmur: diastolic heart sound generated by turbulent blood flow across the mitral valve; caused by aortic insufficiency, which closes the mitral leaflets

ball-in-cage valve: prosthetic heart valve characterized by a caged ball that moves with ventricular pressure to open and close an orifice

bell: cup-shaped portion of the stethoscope that's best suited for listening to low-pitched sounds

bileaflet valve: (1) prosthetic heart valve characterized by two small wings that control blood flow; (2) mitral valve

binaural headpiece: stethoscope headpiece that supplies sounds to both ears simultaneously

blowing: term used to describe a continuous murmur sound like the sound of air passing through pursed lips

booming: term used to describe a deep, resonant heart sound that's sudden and percussive

bronchial circulation: oxygenated blood that arises from the aorta or subclavicular artery and supplies the tracheobronchial tree with oxygen and nutrients

bundle of His: small band of specialized cardiac muscle fibers located in the intraventricular septum that relay atrial electrical impulses to the ventricles

capillary hydrostatic pressure: fluid pressure within the capillary system that, when elevated, leads to fluid extravasation out of the capillary system into the interstitium

cardiac cycle: sequence of events (systole and diastole) that enables the heart to receive and pump blood

cardiac output: quantity of oxygenated blood pumped through the body by the heart, usually expressed in liters per minute; computed as stroke volume × heart rate

cardiac tamponade: heart compression caused by effusion or collection of fluid in the pericardium, resulting in decreased cardiac output

cervical venous hum murmur: murmur caused by rapid downward blood flow through the jugular veins in the lower part of the neck

chordae tendineae: tendinous cords that connect each cusp of the two atrioventricular valves to appropriate papillary muscles in the ventricles

click: short heart sound; also, another term for a midsystolic sound that occurs when a prolapsed mitral valve's leaflet and chordae tendineae tense

click-murmur syndrome: condition in which a click is followed by a murmur, as in mitral valve prolapse syndrome

closing click: heart sound generated by valve closure; heard with all prosthetic valves regardless of their type or position

coarctation of the aorta: localized aortic malformation characterized by deformity of the aortic media and causing severe narrowing of the aortic lumen

compliance: tissue's or organ's ability to yield to pressure without disruption; commonly used to describe the distensibility of an air- or fluid-filled organ, such as the heart or lungs

conduction system: specialized cardiac cells and fibers that initiate or relay electrical impulses, stimulating the heart muscle to contract

configuration: shape of a murmur's sound as recorded on a phonocardiogram; one of the characteristics used to describe murmurs

constrictive pericarditis: inflammation of the pericardium that leads to thickening and possible calcification of the pericardial sac, resulting in impaired diastolic filling, inflow stasis, or a constrictive effect

continuous murmur: murmur that begins in systole and persists, without interruption, through S_2 into diastole

contractile cell: one of the myocardial cells that contract to start systole; these cells depolarize and repolarize by means of ion flow

cor pulmonale: heart disease caused by pulmonary hypertension secondary to disease of the lung or its blood vessels, resulting in hypertrophy of the right ventricle

crepitation: crackling sound that resembles the sound made by rubbing hair between two fingers

crescendo: term used to describe the configuration of a murmur that increases in intensity

crescendo-decrescendo: term used to describe the configuration of a murmur that rises in intensity and then fades

cusp: one of the triangular segments of a cardiac valve or one of the semilunar segments of the aortic or pulmonic valve

dampened: diminished sound intensity or amplitude; term used to describe sounds

decrescendo: term used to describe the configuration of a murmur that decreases in intensity

depolarization: movement of sodium ions into a contractile cell, creating a positive charge inside the cell

diamond-shaped murmur: crescendo-decrescendo murmur

diaphragm: primary muscle of respiration, which separates the thoracic and abdominal cavities; also the part of the stethoscope used to auscultate for high-pitched sounds

diastole: expansion of the ventricles occurring in the interval between S_2 and S_1; relaxation of the heart muscle causes the heart to fill with blood during this part of the cardiac cycle

diffuse: widely distributed; not localized

dilation of pulmonic valve ring: expansion of a valve aperture; a dilated pulmonic valve can contribute to a Graham Steell murmur

dull percussion note: deadened, or nonresonant, sound heard when a solid organ or dense body part is percussed

duration: length of time a heart or breath sound is heard; one of the six characteristics used to describe heart sounds

dynamic obstruction: blocked outflow from one of the heart's chambers that can be demonstrated only during myocardial contraction or systole

early diastolic aortic insufficiency: blood backflow from the aorta that occurs early in diastole, when the ventricle is resting and filling with oxygenated blood

ectopic beats: arrhythmic heartbeats arising from places other than the heart's normal pacemaker, the sinoatrial node

edema: excessive accumulation of fluid in intercellular tissue spaces of the body

ejection sound: sound caused by the opening of a stenotic aortic or pulmonic valve, usually occurring early in systole

ejection velocity: measure of the speed of blood flow

epicardial pacing: regulation of the rate of heart muscle contraction by an artificial cardiac pacemaker stimulating the heart through electrical leads attached to the heart surface

frequency: pitch of a breath sound measured in hertz

functional murmur: benign murmur that doesn't impair heart function

gallop rhythm: triple rhythms; the S_1, S_2, S_3 sequence, the S_4, S_1, S_2 sequence, or both, sounds like a horse's gallop

Graham Steell's murmur: pulmonic insufficiency murmur caused by pulmonic hypertension and pulmonic valve ring dilation

heart failure: clinical syndrome caused by left- or right-sided heart dysfunction; left-sided heart failure results in pulmonary edema and breathlessness; right-sided heart failure results in liver congestion, increased venous pressure, and peripheral edema

high-output condition: physiologic state that causes or results in increased cardiac output

holodiastolic: pertaining to the entire diastole; used to describe a murmur that persists throughout diastole

holosystolic: pertaining to the entire systole; used to describe a murmur that persists throughout systole

holosystolic mitral insufficiency: blood backflow caused by an incompetent mitral valve that can be heard throughout systole

hyperinflation: overinflation of the lung that occurs with air trapping in obstructive lung diseases such as emphysema

hypertrophic cardiomyopathy: narrowing or constriction of the left ventricle's subaortic region caused by tissue enlargement in that area; also known as *idiopathic hypertrophic subaortic stenosis;* this condition can be a cause of subvalvular aortic stenosis

hypertrophy: enlargement or overgrowth of an organ, or part of an organ, caused by an increase in the size of its constituent cells

hypoxemia: abnormally low oxygen tension in arterial blood

idiopathic: of unknown cause

incompetent valve: heart valve that can't perform its functions because of congenital defects, disease, or trauma

infective endocarditis: inflammation of the endocardium caused by infection with microorganisms (bacteria or fungi); primarily affects the heart valves

inferior vena cava: venous trunk for the lower extremities and the pelvic and abdominal viscera

intensity: degree of loudness; one of six characteristics used to describe heart sounds

intercostal muscle: one of the muscles found between the ribs; internal and external intercostal muscles help stabilize and expand or lower the rib cage with ventilation

internodal pathway: one of the fibers connecting the small masses of tissue that transmit the electrical impulses setting the heart's rate and rhythm

interventricular septum: dividing wall between the heart's ventricles

intrapleural pressure: relative pressure that occurs between the pleurae; negative pressure occurs during inspiration; positive pressure occurs during expiration

intrinsic: naturally occurring electrical stimulus from within the heart's conduction system

ischemia: decreased blood supply to a body organ or tissue

isovolumic contraction: initial period in early systole when the atrioventricular and semilunar valves are closed and intraventricular pressures rise but blood hasn't yet been ejected from the ventricles

isovolumic relaxation: brief period in early diastole when the atrioventricular (AV) and semilunar valves are closed, just before the AV valves open and passive filling of the ventricles begins

leaflet: structure resembling a small leaf, especially a heart valve's cusps

left atrial shunt: small amount of deoxygenated blood that returns to the left atrium; normally, this is venous return from bronchial circulation

left bundle-branch block: interrupted conduction through the fiber that activates the left ventricle, resulting in a prolonged or abnormal QRS complex

left lateral recumbent position: position that brings the heart's apex closer to the chest wall for auscultation; the patient lies on his left side, with his right knee and thigh drawn up to his chest

left-sided heart failure: inability of the left ventricle to pump blood adequately, causing decreased cardiac output, which results in pulmonary congestion and edema

left ventricular decompensation: failure of the left ventricle's myocardium to contract and maintain adequate cardiac output

left ventricular hypertrophy: enlargement of the left ventricle's myocardium, which can result in reduced or abnormal ventricular functioning

left ventricular outflow obstruction: stenosis or other blockage preventing flow of oxygenated blood from the left ventricle into the aorta

left ventricular pressure overload: increased pressure within the left ventricle that impairs its ability to function normally; commonly caused by excessively elevated systemic blood pressure

left ventricular volume overload: excessive volume within the left ventricle that causes it to become distended and impairs its ability to function normally

location: site at which a breath or a heart sound can be auscultated

mediastinal crunch: heart sound created by heart movement against air in the mediastinum; also known as *Hamman's sign*

mediastinum: tissues separating the two lungs, between the sternum and the vertebral column and from the thoracic inlet to the diaphragm; contains the heart and its vessels, the trachea, esophagus, thymus, lymph nodes, and other organs and tissues

middiastolic aortic insufficiency: turbulent backward blood flow through the aorta into the left ventricle occurring midway between S_2 and S_1

middiastolic click: click heard midway between S_2 and S_1 in the cardiac cycle; usually associated with a stenotic or rigid atrioventricular valve

midsystolic ejection murmur: crisp, high-frequency sound resulting from a stenotic aortic or pulmonic valve opening in systole

mitral insufficiency: turbulent backward blood flow from the left ventricle into the left atrium caused by the mitral valve's inability to close completely

mitral stenosis: mitral valve narrowing or constriction

mitral valve: tissue folds that, when closed, prevent blood flow from the left ventricle to the left atrium; also called the *bicuspid valve*

mitral valve prolapse: mitral valve bulging from the proper position back toward the left atrium during systole; it can result in mitral insufficiency

murmur: sound heard during auscultation that results from vibrations produced by blood moving within the heart and adjacent blood vessels; may be benign or abnormal

myocardial infarction: tissue death in the heart's muscle; usually caused by inadequate coronary artery perfusion

myocardium: heart wall, comprised of cardiac muscle tissue

nonejection click: click caused by a valve that isn't associated with movement of blood through or across the valve; commonly used to describe the click of mitral valve prolapse

normal sinus rhythm: normal physiologic heart rhythm originating in the sinoatrial node; usually considered to be 60 to 100 beats per minute

opening click: opening sound created by some prosthetic heart valves or by a diseased valve

opening snap: sound created by mitral valve leaflets that have become stenotic or abnormally narrowed but that are still somewhat mobile

oscillation: vibration, fluctuation

P_2: pulmonic component of S_2

papillary muscle: muscular protrusion, or projection, in the ventricles that attaches to and regulates the atrioventricular valves by way of the chordae tendineae

parenchyma: functioning cells of an organ that distinguish or determine the primary organ function

patent ductus arteriosus: abnormal channel connecting the pulmonary artery to the descending aorta; results in arterial blood recirculation through the lungs

perfusion: blood flow to or through an organ or tissue supplied by the blood vessels

pericardial fluid: fluid in the space between the visceral and parietal layers of the pericardium

pericardial friction rub: characteristic high-pitched friction noise created by inflamed or dry pericardial surfaces rubbing together

pericardial knock: S_3 associated with constrictive pericarditis

pericarditis: inflammation of the pericardium

pericardium: two-layer fibrous sac that surrounds the heart and the roots of the great vessels

peripheral: toward the outer boundary or perimeter; not central

peripheral vascular resistance: resistance to the passage of blood through the small blood vessels, especially the arterioles, caused by friction between the blood and the blood vessel wall

phonocardiogram: graphic record of heart sounds and murmurs, including pulse tracings, produced by phonocardiography

physiologic S_3: S_3 that isn't associated with an abnormal condition; commonly found in young individuals

pitch: a tone's vibration or frequency, measured in cycles per second as sound amplitude; subjectively described as high, medium, or low

plateau-shaped murmur: murmur in which intensity is the same, or flat, throughout its duration

pleurae: thin, serous membranes that surround the lungs (visceral pleura) and line the thoracic cavity's inner walls (parietal pleura)

pleural crackle: loud, grating sound caused by inflamed or damaged pleurae

pleural effusion: abnormal accumulation of fluid between visceral and parietal pleurae

pleural friction rub: sound created by friction between the parietal and visceral pleurae surrounding the lungs

pneumothorax: accumulation of air within the pleural cavity

point of maximal impulse: chest wall site where the heartbeat can be seen or felt most strongly; commonly located over the heart's apex

porcine valve: prosthetic heart valve made from swine (pig) products

preload: stretching force exerted on the ventricular muscle by the blood it contains at the end of diastole

pressure gradient: difference in pressure between two regions

PR interval: time between atrial depolarization and ventricular depolarization, as recorded on the electrocardiogram; the PR interval begins at the onset of the P wave and lasts until the onset of the QRS complex; ordinarily, atrial contraction occurs during the PR interval

prosthetic valve: artificial heart valve; ball-in-cage, bileaflet, porcine, and tilting-disk are four types

pulmonary artery: blood vessel leading from the right ventricle to the lungs

pulmonary artery dilation: expansion or stretching of the pulmonary artery beyond its normal dimensions

pulmonary circulation: blood pumped by the right ventricle into the pulmonary artery that circulates through the pulmonary capillary beds, where gas exchange occurs; the oxygenated blood is carried to the left atrium via the pulmonary veins

pulmonary edema: excessive accumulation of fluid within the lung

pulmonary hypertension: increased blood pressure within the pulmonary circulation

pulmonary vein: one of four veins that return oxygenated blood from the lungs to the heart's left atrium

pulmonic ejection sound: high-pitched click commonly created by the opening of a stenotic pulmonic valve; it's the only right-sided heart sound whose intensity increases during expiration and decreases during inspiration

pulmonic insufficiency: abnormal condition of backward blood flow across the pulmonic valve during diastole

pulmonic stenosis: narrowing or constriction of the pulmonic valve or the region just above or below the valve

pulmonic valvular stenosis: narrowing or constriction of the pulmonic valve

Purkinje fibers: modified cardiac muscle cells found beneath the endocardium; they are part of the heart's electrical impulse-conducting system

P wave: part of the electrocardiogram tracing that represents atrial depolarization

QRS complex: electrocardiogram waves representing the spread of electrical impulses from the bundle branches to the ventricular muscle; the QRS complex corresponds to ventricular depolarization

quality: heart sound characteristic determined by a combination of the sound's frequencies; one of six characteristics used to describe heart sounds; a sound's quality may be described as sharp, dull, booming, snapping, blowing, harsh, or musical

radiation: spread of a heart sound beyond its area of origin

regurgitant murmur: sound created by turbulent backward blood flow through an incompetent heart valve

repolarization: movement of calcium ions into the cell and potassium ions out of the cell, followed by the extrusion of sodium and calcium ions from the cell and the restoration of potassium ions into the cell by the sodium-potassium pump

resistance: force that hinders motion; hindrance or impedance

resonance: sound quality produced by percussing structures or cavities that radiate sound vibrations and energy

respiratory cycle: one complete cycle of inspiration and expiration

rheumatic heart disease: valvular abnormalities that are a sequela of rheumatic fever; most commonly, mitral, tricuspid, or aortic stenosis and insufficiency

right bundle-branch block: interrupted conduction through the fiber that activates the right ventricle, resulting in a prolonged QRS complex

right-sided heart failure: inability of the right ventricle to continue functioning properly

right-sided S_3: heart sound caused by a noncompliant right ventricle and high right atrial pressure; it's heard in patients with cor pulmonale, pulmonary embolism, right-sided heart failure secondary to mitral stenosis with left-sided heart failure or pulmonary hypertension, and severe tricuspid insufficiency

right-sided S_4: S_4 generated in the right ventricle; commonly heard in conditions that create pressures greater than 100 mm Hg in that ventricle; it may accompany such conditions as pulmonic stenosis, pulmonary hypertension, or sudden tricuspid insufficiency

right ventricular outflow obstruction: stenosis, embolus, or other blockage preventing flow of deoxygenated blood from the right ventricle into the pulmonary artery

S_1: first heart sound; produced by closure of the mitral and tricuspid valves

S_2: second heart sound; produced by closure of the aortic and pulmonic valves

S_3: third heart sound; created by vibrations caused by the rapid, passive filling of the ventricles; S_3 is abnormal in adults older than age 20; the cadence is similar to the word "Tennessee"

S_4: fourth heart sound; generated by stretching and filling of a ventricle during late diastole; associated with atrial contraction; the cadence is similar to the word "Kentucky"

semilunar valves: heart valves between the ventricles and the pulmonary artery and aorta

shunting: abnormal communication between the high-pressure arterial system and the low-pressure venous system

sinoatrial node: small mass of tissue at the junction of the superior vena cava and the right atrium, which triggers the electrical impulses that begin the cardiac cycle

snap: short, sharp heart sound associated with sudden closing or opening of a heart valve

stenosis: narrowing or constriction of a passage, specifically a heart valve or region around the outflow tract of any of the heart's chambers

sternal border: auscultatory area along and to either side of the sternum

stethoscope: instrument used in auscultation; usually consists of a diaphragm and a bell, which are connected to one or two tubes leading to a binaural headpiece and earpieces

stroke volume: amount of blood pumped during each ventricular contraction

subcutaneous emphysema: presence of air or gas in the tissues beneath the skin; it results in crackling or crepitus when touched

subvalvular aortic stenosis murmur: murmur caused by a left ventricular outflow obstruction below the aortic valve

subvalvular pulmonic stenosis: narrowing or constriction of the region below the pulmonic valve

subvalvular pulmonic stenosis murmur: murmur caused by a right ventricular outflow obstruction below the pulmonic valve

summation gallop: S_4 that occurs simultaneously with S_3, thus sounding louder

superior vena cava: major vein that drains blood from the upper half of the body, beginning below the right costal cartilage and continuing to the right atrium

supine: lying on the back, face up

supravalvular aortic stenosis murmur: murmur caused by left ventricular outflow obstruction above the aortic valve

supravalvular pulmonic stenosis: narrowing or constriction of the region above the pulmonic valve

supravalvular pulmonic stenosis murmur: murmur caused by a right ventricular outflow obstruction above the pulmonic valve

systemic hypertension: condition in which the patient has a higher-than-normal overall blood pressure

systole: ventricular contraction that ejects blood into the arterial system; the left ventricle ejects into the aorta, and the right ventricle ejects into the pulmonary artery

systolic crescendo murmur: heart sound that begins as a faint sound, then rises in volume; occurs during the ventricular contraction phase of the cardiac cycle

systolic ejection murmur: murmur heard in systole that's caused by turbulent blood flow as the right or left ventricle ejects blood; it can be an innocent murmur

systolic insufficiency murmur: sound created by turbulent backward blood flow from either the mitral or tricuspid valve during the ventricular contraction phase of the cardiac cycle

T_1: tricuspid component of S_1

thoracic cavity: space within the rib cage that begins at the clavicle and ends at the diaphragm

thorax: bony structure that encloses the thoracic cavity, protecting the heart, lungs, and great vessels

thrill: abnormal tremor felt on palpation that accompanies some vascular or cardiac murmurs

tilting-disk valve: prosthetic heart valve characterized by a disk that tilts with ven

tricular pressure to open and close the valvular opening

tracheobronchial tree: portion of the airway that begins at the larynx and ends at the terminal bronchioles; also known as the *lower airway*

tricuspid insufficiency: tricuspid valve incompetence during systole, which allows turbulent backward, or regurgitant, blood flow into the right atrium

tricuspid stenosis: narrowing or constriction of the tricuspid valve

tricuspid valve: heart valve between the right atrium and right ventricle

turbulence: disturbed or irregular airflow; can be caused by rapid flow rates or variations in air pressures and velocities

T wave: part of the electrocardiogram tracing that represents ventricular repolarization

Valsalva's maneuver: attempt to exhale forcibly with the glottis closed

ventricular ejection: ventricular contraction that sends blood into the arterial system; called *systole* in the cardiac cycle

ventricular fibrillation: chaotic, disorganized pattern of electrical impulses coming from multiple ectopic sites in the ventricles; an arrhythmia that produces no effective ventricular mechanical activity and no cardiac output

ventricular filling: ventricular relaxation and expansion that allows blood to enter; called *diastole* in the cardiac cycle

ventricular outflow obstruction: blockage in the valve or vessel that carries blood out of one of the heart's ventricles

ventricular septal defect: opening in the septum between the ventricles; usually represents a congenital abnormality

ventricular tachycardia: rapid heart rate originating from one or more ectopic foci in the ventricle

Selected references

Altman, C.A., et al. *Pediatric Cardiac Auscultation CD-ROM.* Philadelphia: Lippincott Williams & Wilkins, 2001.

Bickley, L.S. *Bates' Guide to Physical Examination and History Taking,* 8th ed. Philadelphia: Lippincott Williams & Wilkins, 2002.

Blaufox, M.D. *An Ear to the Chest: An Illustrated History of the Evolution of the Stethoscope.* Boca Raton: CRC-Press, 2002.

Bloch, A., et al. "Should Functional Cardiac Murmurs be Diagnosed by Auscultation or by Doppler Echocardiography?" *Clinical Cardiology* 24(12):767-69, December 2001.

Cardiovascular Care Made Incredibly Easy. Philadelphia: Lippincott Williams & Wilkins, 2005.

Chizner, M.A. "The Diagnosis of Heart Disease by Clinical Assessment Alone," *Current Problems in Cardiology* 26:285-379, 2001.

ECG Interpretation Made Incredibly Easy, 3rd ed. Philadelphia: Lippincott Williams & Wilkins, 2004.

Friedman, A.W. *Clinical Cardiology Skills: EKG and Auscultation.* Philadelphia: American College of Physicians, 2004.

Hanna, I.R., and Silverman, M.E. "A History of Cardiac Auscultation and Some of its Contributors," *American Journal of Cardiology* 90(3):259-67, August 2002.

Illustrated Manual of Nursing Practice, 3rd ed. Philadelphia: Lippincott Williams & Wilkins, 2002.

Medical-Surgical Nursing Made Incredibly Easy. Philadelphia: Lippincott Williams & Wilkins, 2004.

Richardson, T.R., and Moody, J.M. "Bedside Cardiac Examination: Constancy in a Sea of Change," *Current Problems in Cardiology* 25(11):783-825, November 2000.

Schneiderman, H. "Cardiac Auscultation and Teaching Rounds: How Can Cardiac Auscultation Be Resuscitated?" *American Journal of Medicine* 110(3):233-35, February 2001.

Shub, C. "Echocardiography or Auscultation? How to Evaluate Systolic Murmurs," *Canadian Family Physician* 49:163-67, February 2003.

Index

i refers to an illustration; t refers to a table.

i refers to an illustration; t refers to a table.

i refers to an illustration; t refers to a table.

i refers to an illustration; t refers to a table.

Notes

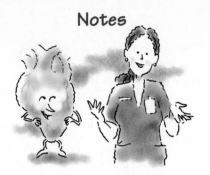

Notes

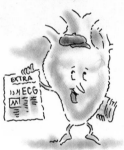

Audio CD cues

Track	Sound		Track	Sound
1, 2	Normal S_1 and S_2 (base of heart)		39, 40	Aortic ejection sound
3	S_1 (mitral area)		41, 42	Midsystolic click
4	S_1 split so M_1 and T_1 can be heard better on expiration (tricuspid area)		43, 44	Innocent systolic ejection murmur
5	S_1 mitral area		45, 46	Supravalvular pulmonic stenosis murmur
6	S_1 split		47, 48	Pulmonic valvular stenosis murmur
7	Abnormal S_1 split		49, 50	Subvalvular pulmonic stenosis murmur
8, 9	S_2 (pulmonic area)		51, 52	Supravalvular aortic stenosis murmur
10, 11	S_2 split during inspiration and expiration		53, 54	Aortic valvular stenosis murmur
12	Increased intensity of P_2		55, 56	Subvalvular aortic stenosis murmur
13	Increased intensity of A_2		57, 58	Tricuspid regurgitation (insufficiency) murmur
14	Diminished A_2		59, 60	Holosystolic mitral regurgitation (insufficiency) murmur
15	S_2 split during inspiration and expiration		61, 62	Acute mitral regurgitation (insufficiency) murmur
16	Paradoxical S_2 split heard during expiration		63	Mitral valve prolapse murmur with click
17	Persistent S_2 split		64	Mitral valve prolapse murmur
18	Persistent S_2 split in pulmonary hypertension		65, 66	Early diastolic aortic regurgitation (insufficiency) murmur
19, 20	Wide, fixed S_2 split		67, 68	Austin Flint murmur
21	Paradoxical S_2 split		69, 70	Graham Steell murmur
22	Fused paradoxical S_2 split		71, 72	Normal pressure pulmonic valve murmur
23, 24	S_3 over mitral area (S_1, S_2, S_3)		73, 74	Mitral stenosis murmur (atrial fibrillation)
25, 26	Abnormal S_3		75	Mitral stenosis murmur (normal sinus rhythm)
27, 28	Pericardial knock		76, 77	Tricuspid stenosis murmur
29, 30	Right-sided S_3		78, 79	Cervical venous hum murmur
31, 32	S_4 (S_4, S_1, S_2)		80, 81	Patent ductus arteriosus murmur
33	Summation gallop		82	Aortic prosthetic valve sound and murmur
34	Right-sided S_4		83	Mitral prosthetic valve sound and murmur
35, 36	Opening snap of mitral valve		84, 85	Pericardial friction rub
37, 38	Pulmonic ejection sound		86, 87	Mediastinal crunch